Sex and the Overweight: How Plus-Sized Individuals Can Find Happiness, Best Sex Positions, and a Fulfilling Sexual Journey

By

Patti W. Nieves

Copyright:

Disclaimer:

The content provided in "Sex and the Overweight: How Plus-Sized Individuals Can Find Happiness, Best Sex Positions, and a Fulfilling Sexual Life" is for informational and educational purposes only. The author, Patti W. Nieves, is not a licensed medical or mental health professional. The information presented in this book is not a substitute for professional advice, diagnosis, or treatment. Readers are encouraged to consult with qualified healthcare or mental health professionals regarding their specific situations.

The author and publisher disclaim any liability, loss, or risk incurred as a consequence, directly or indirectly, of the use and application of any information presented in this book. The reader acknowledges that they are responsible for their own decisions regarding their health, well-being, and sexual practices. By reading this book, the reader agrees to hold harmless the author and publisher from any consequences or actions arising from the use of the information provided.

Every effort has been made to ensure the accuracy of the information presented in this book. However, the author and publisher do not assume and hereby disclaim any liability to any party for any loss, damage, or disruption caused by errors or omissions, whether such errors or omissions result from negligence, accident, or any other cause.

Any reference to specific brands, products, or services in this book does not imply endorsement or recommendation by the author or publisher. The views and opinions expressed in this book are solely those of the author and do not necessarily reflect the official policy or position of any other individual, organization, or entity.

About the Author: Patti W. Nieves

Patti W. Nieves is a committed content developer in the field of sexuality and a fervent supporter of sexual fulfillment. Patti contributes a distinct viewpoint to the conversation on sex and body positivity because of her dedication to creating positive narratives around intimate well-being.

Patti devotes her efforts as a proponent of sexual fulfillment to challenging social standards that frequently obstruct people from having meaningful sexual relationships, particularly those who are plus-sized. Her art reveals a profound comprehension of the complexities of negotiating relationships, pleasure, and self-acceptance in a society that occasionally sets unattainable expectations.

Patti's path as a sexuality content provider is distinguished by her dedication to empowerment and education. She provides her knowledge, counsel, and nuanced viewpoints across a variety of platforms in an effort to promote candid discussions regarding a range of sexual experiences. Her writings demonstrate her commitment to inclusivity and her understanding that everyone deserves to have a happy and fulfilled sexual life, regardless of size.

Patti W. Nieves takes readers on a journey to a world where having a talk about sex is acceptable without passing judgment and where accepting oneself is essential to forming happy relationships. Patti hopes to create a world where everyone may find happiness and fulfillment in their own special way by empowering others to accept their bodies, wants, and pleasures through her activism and content creation.

Table of Contents

Introduction

This book bravely explores the complex world of plus-sized sexual relationships in a society that frequently upholds limited notions of beauty. It aims to demolish assumptions, promote body acceptance, and offer a thorough manual on how people with a variety of body types can develop fulfilling sexual relationships in addition to finding pleasure. This book explores the complex path of accepting one's body and creating incredibly satisfying relationships, covering everything from cultural preconceptions to discovering the finest sex positions.

Unrealistic standards have long defined the prevailing culture narrative surrounding body image, negatively affecting people who identify as plus-sized. The book begins by recognizing the widespread impact of society's opinions and the difficulties they present for those who want to accept their bodies. By breaking down these stereotypes, we hope to give plus-sized people the confidence to take back control of their story and create a paradigm shift in favor of acceptance and self-love.

Building on this base, the book explores the emotional terrain, digging into the most important aspects of social pressure and self-confidence. It gives people doable tactics to strengthen their sense of self-worth, giving them a path to overcome criticism from others and develop an optimistic outlook. By attending to mental well-being, we enable plus-sized people to set out on a path that leads not only to happiness but also the fulfillment of their emotional and sexual desires.

The primary concern of this book is the pursuit of happiness, which goes beyond what society considers to be acceptable. The importance of self-love is emphasized in the book, and pursuing activities and passions that lead to a sense of fulfillment is encouraged. People are led towards a path of self-discovery and are able to create an identity that surpasses social norms by turning the focus inside.

Sexual relationships require effective communication, and the book includes a section devoted to encouraging candid conversations with partners. People can build a foundation of understanding and trust by addressing their fears and insecurities, which fosters an atmosphere that is favorable to both emotional and physical closeness.

By offering information on the ideal sex positions for people of plus size, the investigation dives even deeper into the physical domain. A section, which emphasizes comfort, enjoyment, and diversity, seeks to debunk myths and stereotypes while providing helpful advice to improve the sexual experiences of plus-sized people and their partners.

The book broadens its focus on the larger picture of a satisfying sexual life as it gets closer to the finish. From the value of closeness to the incorporation of diversity and ingenuity, the story aims to offer a comprehensive viewpoint on developing a fulfilling and varied sexual experience for people of plus-size.

Defining How Plus-Sized Individuals Should Explore Sexual Relationships

In a world where norms are frequently set by society, exploring connections with others for people who identify as plus-sized is an important and vital undertaking. In order to reshape society perspectives, demolish prejudices, and promote a deeper awareness of the complexity surrounding the romantic and sexual experiences of persons who identify as plus-sized, we attempt to express the substance of this exploration in this book.

The phrase "plus-sized" itself may imply things that unintentionally support the maintenance of unattainable beauty standards. In order to begin this investigation, the conversation around sexual relationships and body image must be redefined. It is a sophisticated exploration of the emotional, psychological, and social factors that impact the relationship lives of people who identify as plus-sized rather than just a physical assessment.

People's perceptions are frequently distorted by the cultural lens, which can lead to an environment where people feel pressured to meet stringent standards of beauty. In an effort to dispel these social myths, this book promotes an honest and open discussion about the difficulties plus-sized people encounter while attempting to build meaningful relationships. We acknowledge that the exploration of sexual relationships is a journey towards self-acceptance, understanding, and eventually a redefining of what defines a fulfilling relationship, going beyond a simple search for physical connection.

Understanding how cultural norms affect one's perception of one's body and sense of worth becomes increasingly important as we continue this investigation. Through questioning these conventions, the book hopes to free plus-sized people from the chains of outside expectations and create a space where genuine connections and respect can be the foundation of their relationships.

Furthermore, dispelling myths about plus-sized people's desirability, attractiveness, and sexual prowess is essential to exploring sexual interactions for them. We lay the groundwork for debunking falsehoods and advancing a more inclusive narrative that values a range of bodies and experiences by defining this investigation.

This book is an invitation to question assumptions and promote a critical analysis of what it means for people who identify as plus-sized to be in intimate relationships. We hope that by defining this exploration, we will open the door to a conversation that is more inclusive, understanding, and compassionate and that celebrates the complexity of various bodies and the deep beauty found in genuine connections between people.

Overcoming Social Obstacles to Achieve Happiness and Sexual Fulfillment

Social judgments and preconceptions frequently weave a shadow in the complicated labyrinth of human interactions, affecting how people negotiate the domains of sex and happiness. This path becomes especially difficult for those who are overweight because they have to deal with cultural obstacles and prejudices that portray them as outsiders in the story of close relationships and personal fulfillment. The goal of this book is to raise awareness of the significant barriers that overweight people must overcome in order to achieve sexual pleasure and happiness.

Stereotypes about body image are frequently amplified and reinforced by the cultural lens, which is fashioned by frequently unattainable beauty standards. The impact on those who don't fit the mold is evident and affects many facets of their lives, particularly when it comes to sexual relationships. The first step is to acknowledge these societal issues, which foster an atmosphere in which people who are overweight may feel judged, scrutinized, or even unworthy of true happiness.

The widespread misconception that overweight people are somehow less attractive or less capable of having satisfying sexual lives is one of the core issues this book explores. These misconceptions diminish the value of intimate relationships and emotional ties in addition to contributing to body shaming. By drawing attention to these difficulties, we hope to analyze the damaging myths that support prejudice and obstruct overweight people's ability to form real connections.

Furthermore, the pressure from society to live up to predetermined standards of attractiveness can cause unfavorable self-perceptions to be internalized. The combination of external prejudices and self-stigmatization makes it difficult to accept one's physique and find pleasure. This book explores the psychological effects of these stereotypes and highlights how important it is to go above and beyond what society expects in order to achieve true self-love and satisfaction.

The book aims to debunk the myth that one's physical weight is the only criteria that determines one's eligibility for happiness, love, and fulfillment. By bringing attention to these issues, we hope to give overweight people the confidence to question accepted wisdom, rewrite their own stories, and actively contribute to the creation of a dialogue that affirms the worth and capacity for happiness that each and every person, regardless of size, possesses.

"Sex and the Overweight" is essentially a lighthouse of understanding and liberation. It not only clarifies the difficulties that plus-sized people have in sexual relationships, but it also offers helpful advice, methods, and inspiration for embracing body positivity and living happy, self-discovering, and meaningful lives.

Chapter One: Understanding Sex and the Overweight

It is necessary to explore the complicated interactions between cultural norms, individual perspectives, and the specifics of sexual relationships in order to comprehend sex for people who identify as overweight. This comprehensive investigation aims to unravel the complex issues and obstacles that overweight people encounter when it comes to sexuality. It's a complex process to understand sex for overweight people, one that requires breaking down social conventions, promoting self-acceptance, and demolishing prejudices. Recognizing the various stories included within this investigation will enable us to play a part in a cultural revolution that redefines the standards of meaningful and pleasurable sexual relationships for people of all body types, promotes inclusivity, and supports body positivity.

1. Social Perceptions and Beauty Standards: What is considered desirable or attractive is frequently determined by social norms and beauty standards. People who are overweight may struggle with societal norms that value thinness above all else, which can result in the internalization of unfavorable body images.

These ideas are reinforced by media portrayals, which reinforce preconceptions that associate physical attractiveness with a particular body type. People may feel pressured to live up to inflated expectations as a result, which may negatively impact their self-esteem and confidence.

2. Challenging Stereotypes: A common misconception links being overweight to being less desirable. This oversimplification perpetuates negative myths about attractiveness based only on physical appearance by ignoring the variety of ways people experience and express intimacy.

Another myth holds that those who are overweight could not be good sexual partners. It is essential to analyze this misunderstanding because it downplays the significance of shared closeness, emotional connection, and communication in creating satisfying sexual experiences.

3. Internalized Perceptions and Psychological Effects: Prejudices in society have the potential to cause internalized self-stigmatization, which causes people to develop unfavorable opinions about their own bodies. It is essential to overcome these inner conflicts in order to have a positive self-image and a healthy relationship with one's body.

Internalized beliefs have the power to undermine self-esteem and make someone less inclined to participate honestly in close relationships. Fostering self-assurance and fully accepting one's sexuality require addressing these internal obstacles.

4. Shifting Paradigms: A paradigm shift is encouraging people to value their bodies regardless of what society expects of them by promoting body positivity and self-love.

The cornerstone of developing a pleasant and healthful approach to intimate relationships is accepting one's individual body.

It's essential to acknowledge the variety of body forms and experiences. The idea of a single, universal standard of beauty is undermined by an inclusive approach, which highlights the beauty found in every body.

5. Communication and Relationships: It's critical to communicate well in close relationships. When there is honest communication about needs, wants, and boundaries, partnerships flourish. Establishing a comfortable environment for communication, promoting empathy, and removing any potential fears are beneficial to overweight people.

Creating connections based on understanding and respect for one another helps create a supportive atmosphere. A sense of security and acceptance is fostered when people recognize and value each other's individuality.

1. Analyzing Societal Norms and their Impact on Body Image

Media representations play a major role in the construction and reinforcement of societal norms. A limited notion of beauty is frequently upheld by mainstream media, which marginalizes some body types while idealizing others. The construction of these ideals is aided by movies, fashion photos, and advertisements, which produce a visual narrative that frequently leaves out people with different body types. Perceptions of the perfect body are significantly shaped by cultural norms and customs. Different cultural standards of beauty may influence how people view themselves depending on how closely they adhere to or deviate from these norms.

A comprehensive analysis of societal standards and their effects on body image demonstrates the significant impact that cultural expectations can have on people's self-perceptions. This full review explores the ways that cultural norms impact body image, the effects that result from these influences, and the strategies that could be used to promote a better relationship between people and their bodies.

1. Establishment of Social Norms

The process of societal norm creation is complex and dynamic, with strong roots in historical, cultural, and media influences. Let's now examine how these conventions came to be and how they influence how people view their bodies and what constitutes beautiful.

1. Media Portrayals: The media's constant idealization of particular body types—often slender and toned—is a major source of societal norms. These norms are cultivated by advertisements, fashion magazines, and entertainment media, which provide a visual standard to which people are expected to adhere. The widespread use of picture manipulation tools presents impossible expectations of perfection and further distorts reality. Even though Photoshopped photographs are far from the natural diversity of human bodies, they contribute to

the construction of an aspirational style that feeds into society norms.

2. Cultural ideas: Historical contexts, where various eras have honored differing ideas of beauty, are the deepest source of societal norms. For instance, larger forms were valued in Renaissance art, but modern standards frequently favor a more slender build. The mutable character of society norms is partly due to these historical changes. Different historical, geographic, and cultural contexts have impacted different societies' conceptions of beauty. By contrasting these disparate values, the author highlights the arbitrary character of society norms and shows that there is no one set standard.

3. Social Comparisons: The tendency of humans to judge themselves against others is a major factor in the development of society standards. Social comparisons serve as a means of reinforcing and maintaining norms as people see and internalize the perceived societal ideal. As social media usage increases and people are exposed to

well chosen photos that might not accurately represent reality, social comparisons become more intense. Through their online persona, influencers and celebrities—who are sometimes regarded as idealized representations of beauty—play a vital role in influencing society norms.

4. Consumerism and Market Forces: Economic forces and the media both have an impact on societal standards. Certain body stereotypes are used by the fashion, beauty, and fitness industries to fuel consumerism. Narrow beauty standards can be upheld and sustained by financial interests. More people are realizing these days that diversity is a selling point. A growing number of businesses have begun to include more varied representatives after realizing the financial advantages of catering to a wider spectrum of customers.

Recognizing the societal norms' flexibility and their impact on people's views of beauty requires an understanding of how they are formed. Given how these norms have changed over time and across cultural and historical settings, cultivating diversity, challenging constrained norms, and forming social ideals all require a more comprehensive and conscious approach.

2. Effect on Body Image

People internalize beauty standards from an early age as a result of internalizing society norms. People's internalization shapes their self-perception of their bodies, forming a prism through which they assess their value and desirability. Social norms create a culture of comparison in which people evaluate themselves against the ideal they see in society. Constant comparison can cause negative body image development, feelings of inadequacy, and unhappiness.

Social standards have a significant impact on body image, affecting how people see themselves and their mental and emotional health. Let us look at the complex ways in which cultural norms influence how people perceive their bodies and the effects that this might have on them.

1. Internalization of Beauty Ideals: From an early age, people internalize society norms, especially those pertaining to body image. People's self-concepts get ingrained with specific body ideals that they are constantly exposed to through media, advertising, and cultural representations. A culture of comparison is fostered by regular exposure to societal values. People may compare these ideals to their own bodies, and when there is a perceived mismatch, it can have a negative effect on body image and lower self-worth.

2. The Formation of Ridiculous Expectations: Beauty standards that are both unreasonable and unachievable are frequently promoted by societal conventions. People may become unhappy in the pursuit of these ideals—which could include particular body types, sizes, or features—because they may want to achieve an appearance that may be at odds with their inherent qualities. The pressure to live up to these expectations can lead to dangerous habits like binge eating, overexercising, or even taking part in risky

behaviors in order to have an unrealistic body image.

3. Cultural and Gender Impact: Beauty standards are shaped by cultural norms, and people may be under various pressures depending on what is expected of them. For example, people's perceptions of their bodies may be affected by the stark differences between Western and Eastern notions of beauty. Gender-specific beauty standards are frequently imposed by societal norms, which have differing effects on men and women. Men may be swayed by ideas of muscularity, whereas women may experience pressures associated with thinness. These gendered expectations add to the complexity of problems with body image.

4. The Influence of the Media on Body Dysmorphic Disorders: Body dysmorphic disorders may arise as a result of long-term exposure to idealized images in the media. People who have body dysmorphia fix their attention on things that they think are wrong with their looks. This can cause them great distress and make it difficult for them to go

about their everyday lives. Emotional problems like eating disorders and anxiety are exacerbated by the inaccurate representation of bodies in the media. Much psychological pain can result from the discrepancy between society standards and perceived reality.

5. Intersectionality and Marginalized Identities: Issues of race, ethnicity, and socioeconomic status overlap with societal norms. People who belong to oppressed groups could experience additional pressures because beauty standards might not be in line with their ethnic or cultural traits. The effects on self-esteem and body image are amplified by this intersectionality.

It takes a careful analysis of the complicated relationships between media portrayals, cultural expectations, and personal experiences to truly understand how society norms affect body image. Understanding the negative impacts of unattainable standards is essential for advancing acceptance, developing a culture that values various bodies, and advancing a more compassionate and inclusive approach to body image.

3. Psychological Repercussions

Body dysmorphia is an emotional disorder marked by an obsession with perceived imperfections in physical appearance. It can be worsened by social pressure to meet social norms. The condition stems from the misalignment of an individual's perception of themselves with the norms of society. People who don't fit in with society's expectations could feel less confident in themselves. Constant exposure to visuals and messaging that uphold an exclusive beauty standard can undermine self-worth and undermine confidence.

Social standards have significant psychological effects on body image, which frequently materialize as a variety of emotional and mental health issues. The following paragraphs looks deeply into the psychological fallout that people could experience from internalizing society norms surrounding body image.

1. Body Dissatisfaction and Low Self-Esteem: A culture of continual comparison is fostered by the widespread impact of societal norms. People who feel that there is a gap between their bodies and what society considers ideal may be unhappy with their bodies for a long time, which lowers their self-esteem. When people internalize unattainable beauty standards, it can result in a poor self-perception where they harshly assess their own bodies based on an ideal that can be impractical or unachievable given their own qualities.

2. Development of Eating Disorders: Eating disorders may arise as a result of societal standards that place an emphasis on a specific body type or size. When people feel pressured to live up to these standards, they may resort to restricted diets, harmful eating patterns, or, on the other hand, binge eating as a coping mechanism. Anorexia nervosa, bulimia nervosa, and binge-eating disorder are examples of eating disorders that have a major psychological impact on mood, cognitive function, and general mental health.

3. The development of body dysmorphic disorder (BDD) might be attributed to the internalization of cultural ideals. BDD sufferers experience distress and decreased functioning as a result of their obsessive emphasis on perceived imperfections in their looks, which may not conform to society's ideals of beauty. Because people with BDD may avoid social situations or engage in repetitive actions to hide or correct perceived imperfections, it can have a major impact on social functioning and general quality of life.

4. Anxiety and Depression: Higher levels of anxiety and depression may result from the pressure to fit in with society's expectations. Mental health issues can be made worse by ongoing concerns about one's looks, fear of being judged, and the emotional cost of falling short of social expectations. Social norms that reinforce negative body image can start a vicious cycle of negative thoughts and emotions that exacerbate anxiety and depressive symptoms.

5. Self-Worth and Identity: When people internalize society norms, they may have identity crises as a result of feeling that their bodies don't fit with society values. Self-worth issues can surface and affect a person's sense of self and social standing. Psychological repercussions also harm interpersonal connections since people may experience difficulties with closeness, trust, and connection, which can impair their capacity to form and maintain healthy relationships.

6.Intersectionality and Extra Stressors: Intersectionality, the confluence of racial, gender, and socioeconomic standards, can exacerbate psychological difficulties. People who belong to marginalized groups could experience additional pressures stemming from cultural expectations, which could result in a more intricate interaction of psychological effects.

The psychological effects of internalizing body image-related cultural norms highlight how critical it is to create a culture that values diversity, body positivity, and more accurate representations of a range of bodies. It emphasizes how crucial it is to provide mental health assistance, have honest conversations, and work together to confront and alter damaging beauty standards in order to lessen the psychological toll that they have on people.

4. Intersectionality and Societal Standards

Questions of race, gender, and socioeconomic class frequently cross paths with societal standards. The socially constructed standards of beauty can disproportionately impact vulnerable populations, making life more difficult for those who don't match the mold.

The term "intersectionality" describes how social categories like race, gender, and class are interrelated and how their overlaps and intersections result in complicated and individual experiences. Intersectionality is essential to understanding how people from different origins may have compounding obstacles as a result of the convergence of distinct social identities while analyzing the influence of societal standards on body image.

1. Differences Across Cultures in Beauty Ideals: Diverse racial and ethnic groups frequently hold different standards of beauty. In this sense, intersectionality refers to the ability of individuals to navigate standards of beauty that are influenced by both cultural norms and racial or ethnic expectations. For example, people's experiences with Eurocentric beauty standards may vary depending on their race.

2. Double Standards: Double standards in terms of ideal body image result from the intersection of gender norms and society expectations. For instance, men may be impacted by the ideals of muscularity, while women may experience pressures connected to thinness. Gender differences in the experiences of body image issues are partly attributed to intersectionality.

3. The Economic and Social Elements: Body image and socioeconomic position are related because people with different

financial situations may have differing access to beauty standards. Socioeconomic considerations can impact the affordability of cosmetic items, fitness regimens, and even the availability of various media depictions.

4. Age and Body Image: Body image ideals and generational differences are related; older generations may have experienced different social norms than younger generations. Different age groups may experience different pressures to conform and change in beauty standards, which can have an impact on how people view their bodies.

5. Sexual Orientation: When discussing intersectionality in relation to sexual orientation, one admits that various people may have different social norms. LGBTQ+ people may have unique obstacles when it comes to ideas of body image that are shaped by both their own communities and general society norms.

6. Disability and Body Image: Because varied bodies are rarely represented in society norms, people with disabilities may have particular difficulties. Intersectionality emphasizes how crucial it is to take accessibility and representation into account when having conversations regarding body image among individuals with disabilities.

7. Stigma and Mental Health: The relationship between mental health and social standards highlights the possibility of additional stigma for those with mental health concerns who struggle with issues related to body image. The psychological effects may worsen when cultural norms and the stigma associated with mental illness collide.

8. Differing Cultural Contexts: Intersectionality emphasizes how cultural relativism is necessary when talking about body image. People from different cultural origins may have different opinions on body image, impacted by their own society norms. Cultural norms and expectations might vary greatly.

Promoting inclusivity and appreciating the range of experiences that people have requires an understanding of intersectionality in the context of cultural norms and body image. Recognizing the complex obstacles encountered by individuals straddling multiple social identities highlights the need of advancing body acceptance that takes into account the complexity of human variety.

5. Encouraging a Positive Body Image

Promoting diversity and inclusivity in representations is essential to cultivating a positive body image. A more inclusive cultural narrative is facilitated by the media, advertising, and other outlets' celebration of a variety of body kinds. By putting in place educational programs that emphasize self-acceptance and body positivity, society standards can be challenged and reshaped.

Crucial components of these programs include giving people the skills to assess media messages critically and building resistance against damaging beauty standards.

A multimodal approach that includes supportive communities, societal changes, and individual self-care is needed to foster a positive body image. Below we look at a thorough guide on methods and projects that encourage a healthy relationship with one's body:

1. Encouraging Media Literacy: Assist people in evaluating media portrayals of attractiveness. Programs for media literacy can educate participants how to analyze the narratives and images that uphold unattainable beauty standards. Promote and assist media that features a range of racial, ethnic, and physical characteristics. Greater visibility of all body types supports a cultural narrative that is more inclusive.

2. Body Positivity Education: Put in place educational initiatives that support self-acceptance and body positivity in schools and communities. Educating people about the value of various bodies and the impractical nature of society's standards of beauty can give them the confidence to question damaging conventions.

3. Deconstructing Stigmas: Recognize and lessen the stigma associated with mental health, with special emphasis on the relationship between mental health and body image. Encourage candid discussions to normalize asking for help when you need it for mental health issues relating to body image.

4. Building Inclusive Environments: Make sure that a variety of body portrayals are shown in public areas, ads, and social media platforms. A sense of belonging is fostered by inclusive imagery for people of different identities, sizes, and shapes. Encourage the availability of fashion and beauty goods that are accessible to people with impairments. Diversity is celebrated and obstacles are broken down with the aid of inclusive design and representation.

5. Promote the use of language that is affirming and positive when talking about one's body. Language matters, and encouraging a vocabulary that embraces individuality instead of upholding unattainable norms might help people have a

positive body image. Put functionality above looks. Honor the abilities of bodies rather than just how they look, placing a focus on resilience, strength, and health.

6. Supportive Community Engagement: Form and assist community organizations that promote self-love and body acceptance. These communities give people a forum to exchange stories, lend support, and encourage group empowerment. Encourage local campaigns that question conventional notions of beauty and foster acceptance. Events, workshops, and art projects can support positive body image and a sense of community.

7. Empowerment Through Education: Offer workshops on self-care practices that emphasize holistic well-being, including mental, emotional, and physical health. Educate individuals on the importance of self-compassion and the role of self-care in promoting a positive body image. Highlight and celebrate individuals who serve as positive role models for body acceptance. Showcase diverse role models from various

fields to demonstrate that success and happiness are not limited by appearance.

8. Family Involvement: Provide resources and guidance for parents to promote body positivity in their children. Encourage conversations about self-esteem, body diversity, and healthy relationships with food and exercise within families. Educate families on media literacy to navigate the impact of societal norms on body image collectively. Promote discussions that challenge unrealistic beauty ideals and reinforce positive values.

9. Inclusive Healthcare Practices: Promote inclusive healthcare procedures that give priority to holistic well-being and take into account a variety of body types. Healthcare professionals ought to receive training on how to sensitively and inclusively handle mental health issues pertaining to body image.

10. Legislation and Policy Advocacy: Promote and back laws that shield people from discrimination on the basis of their body. In

order to promote diversity and challenge negative societal practices, legislation might be extremely important.

11. Therapy and Counseling: Make sure you have access to therapy and counseling services that concentrate on body image issues. Mental health practitioners can offer specialized assistance to people dealing with issues pertaining to body image and social conventions.

12. Social Media Ads Promoting Positivity: Encourage and take part in social media initiatives that support self-love and body positivity. Hashtags and challenges have the power to spread, building an encouraging online community that opposes damaging beauty standards.

13. Integrating the School Curriculum: Encourage the inclusion of lessons on body positivity in school curricula. Early on, cultivating a healthy viewpoint can be greatly aided by teaching kids about a variety of body types, the influence of societal norms,

and techniques for developing good body image.

14. Studies and Information Gathering: Encourage and carry out studies on how society norms affect how people feel about their bodies, with an emphasis on intersectionality. Evidence-based actions and policies can be informed by thorough data collecting.

It takes a team effort from individuals, communities, organizations, and governments to promote a positive body image. Society may help to create a culture that loves and embraces the diversity of bodies, fostering good self-perception and well-being for everyone, by combining advocacy, education, and supportive programs.

6. Self-Reflection

It is empowering to support people in reflecting on themselves and challenging social conventions. Being conscious of how outside factors affect one's self-perception enables people to actively reject unattainable ideals and adopt a more true to themselves self-image. Creating communities that prioritize support and inclusion can bring people a feeling of community. Redefining beauty standards and questioning social conventions as a group helps create a society that is more caring and inclusive.

Developing a good body image and escaping cultural conventions that could lead to unattainable beauty standards require individual empowerment. The following are essential tactics that people can use to empower themselves and cultivate a positive relationship with their bodies:

1. Introspection and Awareness: Regularly reflect on yourself to gain insight into your own attitudes around your body image. Engage in mindfulness exercises, such as meditation, to develop a closer relationship with your body and mind.

2. Positive Affirmations: Use affirmations to counter negative self-talk by incorporating them into everyday practices. Pay attention

to affirmations that stress acceptance, love, and gratitude for one's individuality.

3. Set Realistic Goals: Instead of focusing on beauty, set goals for your own mental and physical well-being. Examples of these include physical fitness. Honor accomplishments that support general health and are consistent with personal ideals.

4. Define Beauty on Your Own Terms: Go against what society considers beautiful by defining beauty in accordance with your own principles, assets, and special characteristics. Acknowledge that there is a wide range of appearances and traits that make up the subjective and varied concept of beauty.

5. Positive Self-Expression: Use fashion, artistic outlets, and personal style to show your uniqueness. Choose clothes that fit your body type and give you confidence instead of following trends that don't suit your tastes.

6. Surround Yourself with Positivity: Create a social network of people who encourage one another and appreciate people more for their

contributions and character than for their outward looks. Reduce the amount of time you spend with media that upholds unattainable beauty standards and instead look for content that encourages body positivity.

7. Physical Activity for Well-Being: Don't just focus on exercising for looks; instead, take part in physical activities that make you happy and improve your general well-being. Take part in physical activities that help you develop a healthy relationship with your body, like yoga, dance, or outdoor excursions.

8. Practice Self-Compassion: Develop self-compassion by being nice and understanding to yourself. Recognize that everyone is imperfect and that self-acceptance and growth are possible when one is compassionate toward oneself.

9. Educate Oneself: Gain a deeper understanding of outside influences by studying the effects of society standards on body image. Keep yourself up to date on

research challenging detrimental beauty ideals and body positive initiatives.

10. Seek Professional Support: Speak with counselors or mental health specialists who focus on body image and self-esteem. Expert assistance can offer tailored methods for managing social influences and promoting self-sufficiency.

11. Set Boundaries: Set limits with people or situations that worsen one's perception of one's body. Express your boundaries and personal beliefs in an authoritative manner when it comes to remarks or expectations regarding appearance.

12. Take Part in Advocacy: Take part in initiatives that challenge social standards and promote body positivity. Contribute to broader discussions about body acceptance and a range of beauty standards by drawing on personal experiences.

13. Celebrate Achievements: Honor your own accomplishments, whether they have to do with your career, education, or personal

development. Turn the emphasis from seeking approval from others to acknowledging one's own successes and resiliency.

14. Embrace Individuality: Acknowledge that each person is unique and has their own qualities and strengths. Embrace and appreciate individuality. Embrace authenticity and resist the need to live up to predetermined standards of beauty.

15. Lead by Example: Encourage others by setting an example of genuineness and self-assurance. Be a good role model for friends, family, and peers by encouraging self-determination and accepting different perspectives on what constitutes beauty.

In the context of body image, individual empowerment is taking back control of one's own life, appreciating one's individuality, and cultivating a sense of worth that goes beyond outward appearances. By putting these techniques into practice, people can develop self-love, deal with society demands with fortitude, and support a larger body positive movement.

In conclusion, a detailed grasp of the intricate processes at work is necessary to analyze society norms and how they affect body image. Through acknowledging the processes by which societal norms are established, comprehending their impact on people's mental well-being, and proactively advocating for constructive substitutes, society can strive to cultivate a mindset that honors variety, inclusiveness, and the innate charm present in every physical form.

2. Fostering Body Positivity and Cultivating Healthy Perspectives on Intimacy for Plus-Sized Individuals

To cultivate body positivity and promote a healthy view on relationships for plus-sized people in a world dominated by societal norms and unattainable beauty standards, a paradigm shift is necessary. Let us thoroughly explore the various facets of advocacy in these areas, stressing the importance of dispelling myths, encouraging self-acceptance, and fostering welcoming spaces that honor a range of bodies and romantic partnerships

Questioning Traditional Norms: Advocating for body positivity starts with a basic challenge to cultural conventions that uphold limited definitions of beauty. Deconstructing these ideals and highlighting the fact that attractiveness is not limited to a specific body type is at the heart of this endeavor. Advocates try to change the notion of beauty by promoting varied body shapes in popular culture, advertising, and the media. The intention is to break down the boundaries that set social norms by questioning preconceptions and constructing inclusive representations.

Encouragement of Self-Acceptance: Self-acceptance is an essential concept that must be encouraged in order to empower those who identify as plus-sized. The main goal of advocacy work is to promote authenticity and stress that people of all body types should be able to experience love and closeness. In this effort, stories of self-love become invaluable resources, showcasing people who have accepted their bodies, embracing individuality, and encouraging a sense of self-worth that extends beyond outward appearances.

Knowledge and Consciousness: Education is one area where advocacy is being used to challenge traditional norms regarding intimacy and relationships. Intimacy education—which goes beyond outward appearances and emphasizes the value of communication, emotional connection, and respect for one another—is emphasized. Promoting a more complex definition of desire that incorporates mental and emotional ties, proponents support a larger cultural movement away from appearance-centric standards.

Media Representation: The media is a key area for lobbying efforts since it is essential in forming society perceptions. Proponents campaign for the inclusion of plus-sized people in personal and romantic moments, and inclusive photography becomes a potent tool. Working together with body-positive influencers amplifies messages of inclusivity, reaching a variety of audiences and using alternative narratives to subvert social conventions.

The Lingerie and Fashion Industries' Inclusivity: Important venues for promoting body positivity include the fashion and lingerie industries. Proponents demand inclusive representation and a broad selection of sizes and styles to accommodate people who are plus-sized. Campaigns for inclusive advertising celebrate the sensuality and beauty of varied bodies, encouraging self-expression and empowerment.

Establishing and Strengthening Communities: Building encouraging groups is essential to the body positivity movement. Online forums are designed to be secure places where people who identify as plus-sized may exchange stories, counsel, and encouragement on body positivity and close relationships. Events and courses that take place in person also help to foster conversations openly about healthy intimacy, body image, and self-acceptance.

Training Medical Professionals: The healthcare industry is one of the most important venues for advocacy, and efforts are made to guarantee that healthcare personnel get sensitivity training. Ensuring that people of all body sizes receive inclusive and respectful care is the aim. In the healthcare industry, advocates also strive to dispel myths that could lead to prejudice or discrimination against people who are overweight.

Policy Awareness: Policy efforts to promote diversity and combat structural biases are also considered forms of advocacy. Proposals for anti-discrimination laws are becoming more and more prominent, providing plus-sized people with legal safeguards in a variety of contexts, such as the workplace and public areas. Research-based policy recommendations play a crucial role in creating a cultural landscape that is more inclusive.

Programs for Media Literacy: Giving people the tools they need to be media literate becomes essential to lobbying. Programs for media literacy are designed to give viewers the tools they need to evaluate and challenge the social standards that are portrayed in the media, particularly when it comes to close relationships. Education programs work in conjunction with educational institutions and neighborhood associations to incorporate media literacy instruction that dispels stereotypes and encourages body positivity.

Investigation and Gathering of Data: Research is essential to advocacy activities because it offers empirical backing for the experiences of plus-sized people in close relationships. Advocacy methods, policy suggestions, and evidence-based actions are informed by the data gathered. It turns into an effective instrument for opposing pre existing narratives and encouraging more inclusive portrayals.

Working Together with Mental Health Specialists: Collaborations with mental health specialists are prioritized since advocacy and mental health intersect. One area of focus is to provide therapeutic support that is particular to the issues that plus-sized people encounter around intimacy and body image. Experts in mental health provide workshops and seminars that tackle the relationship between interpersonal well-being and body image.

Parental Instruction and Counseling: Parenting resources are also part of advocacy; they provide parents with advice on how to encourage body positivity and constructive views about intimacy with their kids. Comprehensive sex education reforms are supported, with talks about body diversity and the encouragement of positive relationships for people of all body types included.

It takes a coordinated effort on many fronts to promote body positivity and healthy ideas on intimacy for plus-sized people. Campaigns aim to subvert cultural norms, encourage self-acceptance, and establish welcoming settings that honor a range of bodies and romantic partnerships. By means of education, media portrayal, community development, legislative advocacy, and cooperation with mental health specialists, advocates foster a culture transformation that values the inherent worth and autonomy of every person, regardless of their physical dimensions. It takes a community to move toward inclusivity and body positivity, and as cultural narratives change, there is hope for a world that is more understanding and welcoming of people who identify as plus-sized.

Chapter Two: Overcoming Stereotypes and Embracing Self-Love to Help Plus-Sized People Find Happiness

Plus-sized people may have to navigate a society where limited beauty standards frequently alter people's perceptions of what it means to be happy and healthy. We will look into the path that plus-sized people take to find happiness, stressing the value of self-love, dispelling myths, and encouraging a holistic approach to wellbeing. For plus-sized people, finding happiness is a journey characterized by self-love, confronting prejudices, and a dedication to overall well being.

People who practice self-love, dispel negative stereotypes, and support a holistic approach to health are part of a cultural movement that honors variety and encourages inclusivity. This path aims to change cultural myths in addition to pursuing personal pleasure but also about changing the stories that society tells about itself in order to build a society in which everyone may prosper and feel fulfilled, regardless of size.

Taking Up Self-Love

The cornerstone of achieving happiness for those who are plus-sized is learning to embrace who they are. This entails developing a healthy connection with one's body, acknowledging its individuality, and realizing that value is not based on appearance or size. When people prioritize their own happiness and can resolutely negotiate cultural constraints, self-love becomes a transforming force.

1. Developing a Positive Body Image: People who are plus-sized go on a self-discovery journey, appreciating and appreciating the distinctive features that make them who they are. This entails turning the attention away from what society expects and toward valuing each person's unique qualities, abilities, and capabilities. Mindful self-reflection turns into an effective tool for developing a good body image. In this process, negative thoughts are

acknowledged, contested, and replaced with positive affirmations.

2. Fashion and Self-Expression: Fashion turns into a tool for empowerment and self-expression. It is encouraged for plus-sized people to adopt styles that fit and boost their self-esteem, dispelling misconceptions about what constitutes stylish clothing for various body types. The idea that beauty is sizeless is strengthened by the emergence of body-positive fashion trends. Plus-sized people actively engage in and support these movements, changing the way that people view fashion and self-expression.

Taking on Stereotypes
Overcoming negative social preconceptions that reinforce negative perceptions of people who are plus-sized is necessary to navigate a happy life. Proponents actively work to demolish these prejudices by creating spaces that upend preconceptions and encourage inclusivity.

1. Media Representation: Media portrayals are essential in dispelling stereotypes. In order to break out from the restrictive portrayal of plus-sized people in stereotypical roles, advocates strive to promote various narratives that feature these people in diverse situations. Partnering with media organizations turns into a plan for encouraging uplifting portrayals. Advocates and plus-sized people regularly interact with media outlets to guarantee truthful, powerful representations that support a more inclusive cultural narrative.

2. Educational programs: From an early age, educational programs are essential in dispelling preconceptions. Schools and community groups use body positivity teaching to dispel negative preconceptions and create a more welcoming atmosphere. Giving young people who identify as plus-sized the tools they need to resist social pressures becomes a top goal. The goal of educational initiatives is to cultivate a generation of people who reject stereotypes by instilling self-worth and confidence.

Encouraging a Full Perspective on Well-being

For plus-sized people, finding happiness means going beyond what society thinks and cultivating a whole-person approach to health. This emphasizes that well-being is a comprehensive journey by encompassing physical, mental, and emotional elements.

1. Physical Well-Being: Promoting health at every size takes precedence over reaching a particular body size. Plus-sized people prioritize their general health over meeting social norms by participating in activities that enhance their physical well-being. Advocacy initiatives help build inclusive fitness facilities that serve people of all body types. This dispels myths about exercise and plus-sized people and encourages physical activity as a happy, inclusive pastime.

2. Mental and Emotional Well-Being: People who identify as plus-sized can receive mental health services that acknowledge the connection between emotional well-being and body image. Experts in mental health provide advice on overcoming social

constraints and developing an optimistic outlook. Networks of community support become essential to mental and emotional health. Plus-sized people can share stories, ask for guidance, and find support in online and offline networks as they work towards happiness.

1. Building Self-Confidence and Resilience Against Societal Pressures

A transforming path that enables people to navigate external expectations, appreciate their uniqueness, and create a strong sense of self-worth is building self-confidence and resilience against society pressures. In this investigation, we explore the tactics and mentalities that help people grow resilient and self-assured, allowing them to flourish in the face of social pressure.

It is a dynamic and powerful process to develop resilience and self-confidence in the face of societal pressures. Individuals begin on a transforming journey towards resilience and authentic self-expression by prioritizing personal growth, accessing support networks, setting personal boundaries, accepting positive mindset shifts, and nurturing a deep awareness of their own value. This journey is not about conforming to external expectations but about cultivating an unshakeable belief in one's capabilities, uniqueness, and inherent worth, regardless of societal pressures.

1. Knowing Yourself-Worth

In the complex world of interactions between individuals, knowing oneself comes to play an essential part, particularly for plus-sized people trying to find happiness in the context of sex and society's views of being overweight. It explores the complex interactions that exist between the pursuit of happiness and a sense of self-worth, highlighting the ways in which resilience, fulfilling relationships, and pleasant experiences are all influenced by a strong sense of value within oneself.

When it comes to addressing happiness for plus-sized people in the context of sex and cultural attitudes of overweight, knowing one's own value is key. Recognizing inherent value, accepting individuality, overcoming social stigmas, and cultivating a good self-image are all part of this comprehensive exploration. Plus-sized people develop resilience, confidence, and authenticity via these subtle yet empowering mentality modifications, which pave the road for true satisfaction in close relationships.

Understanding one's own value goes beyond an inward journey to become a potent weapon for subverting social norms, redefining beauty standards, and opening doors for experiences that are affirming and inclusive in the quest for happiness. It is a narrative of empowerment, self-love, and the recognition that happiness in intimate relationships is not dictated by body size but is an inherent right to be claimed and celebrated.

1. Acknowledging Inner Value: The path to self-worth discovery begins with a deep realization of intrinsic value. For plus-sized people trying to find satisfaction in close relationships, this means making a conscious decision to deviate from social norms and

outside measurements. It is a brave admission that one's intrinsic value is a non-negotiable part of one's existence and is not dependent on meeting rigid beauty standards. This change in perspective serves as the foundation for developing self-love and accepting the distinctive traits that give each person intrinsic value.

Acknowledging inherent worth becomes especially relevant when considering the relationship between sex and perceptions of obesity. Realizing that one's value is independent of conforming to established body size norms subverts social constructs that uphold unattainable beauty standards. This shift in perspective enables plus-sized people to pursue pleasure on terms that are genuine and affirming of themselves, and to approach personal encounters with confidence, free from the weight of outside criticism.

2. Embracing Individuality and Body Positivity: Developing a body-positive mindset and accepting one's uniqueness go hand in hand with knowing one's own value.

This transition entails celebrating their bodies for the unique features they possess, which is important for plus-sized people who are navigating happiness, particularly in the context of sex. Choosing to embrace one's uniqueness is a potent act of self-love that promotes confidence and a positive self-perception that transcends societal expectations.

Body positivity challenges prevailing ideas about appearance in personal relationships. Plus-sized people discover that pleasure and desirability are not exclusive benefits only afforded to certain body types, and instead, they learn to value and enjoy their bodies. This change helps to create an environment in which people can have personal experiences free from the burden of social expectations, which in turn promotes feelings of empowerment, liberty, and enjoyment.

3. Overcoming Stereotypes and Stigmas in Society: Knowing oneself to be valuable serves as a strong defense against the prejudices and stigmas that plus-sized people encounter in society, particularly when it comes to sex and the idea of being overweight. It entails an unyielding knowledge that one's value transcends the constrained boundaries of society norms and an unwavering perseverance in the face of external assessments. This change gives people the confidence to question preconceptions and beauty standards, giving them the ability to define their own pleasure.

Overcoming societal stigmas in personal relationships requires navigating happiness free from preconceived preconceptions. Plus-sized people learn to accept their bodies and their worth, realizing that they deserve to be loved, happy, and fulfilled. This change in perspective helps people become more resilient, allowing them to move through private situations with assurance, sincerity, and a profound understanding that their happiness is not contingent on fitting into societal norms.

4. Developing a Positive Self-Image in Intimate Moments: Promoting a positive self-image in intimate moments is closely related to understanding one's own worth. In their quest for sex-related satisfaction, plus-sized people experience a mental transformation that validates their sexual self-assurance. This entails realizing that attractiveness and confidence are innate qualities of an individual's identity rather than being influenced by body size.

This change gives plus-sized people the confidence to fully express their sexuality in close relationships. It promotes the investigation of various sexual expressions, unrestricted by social norms and preconceived ideas. Creating a supportive and affirming atmosphere in which people can experience happiness and fulfillment on their terms is facilitated by cultivating a good self-image during intimate moments.

2. The Transformative Power of Mindset Shifts

The first step in being resilient to societal pressures is to change one's perspective from one of continuous comparison to one of self-celebration. Instead of comparing oneself to other standards, people are advised to recognize their own qualities and accomplishments.

Accepting flaws as a natural aspect of being human is a key component in developing resilience. Acknowledging the impossibility of achieving perfection enables people to adopt a more self-compassionate mindset.

Mindset shifts are transforming agents that challenge society conventions and enable people to embrace a good and gratifying experience in the pursuit of happiness for plus-sized individuals, particularly in the area of sex and intimacy. It explores the nuances of mentality changes and their significant effects on plus-sized people's happiness, self-acceptance, and general well-being in sexual relationships.

1. Adopting a Body-Positive Mentality: For plus-sized people, developing a body-positive perspective is essential to navigate happiness. This calls for a deep change of perspective toward self-love and an understanding of the individuality of one's body. It is recommended for plus-sized people to embrace sensuality at any size in opposition to the limited ideals of beauty that are pushed by society conventions. This mentality change builds self-assurance and destroys the damaging belief that physical attributes are limited to particular body types.

Furthermore, this change involves self-acceptance in close relationships as well as external affirmation. Plus-sized people experience a metamorphosis in which they come to terms with the fact that society does not determine their value or desirability. Instead, accepting one's body in private becomes a powerful gesture of self-love that cultivates a positive self-image that lays the foundation for fulfilling sexual experiences.

2. Overcoming prejudices and Stigmas in Society: Mindset changes are essential in assisting plus-sized people in overcoming prejudices and stigmas in society related to intimacy and body size. By questioning conventional beauty standards, people learn to be resilient against harmful preconceptions and acknowledge the inclusion and diversity of beauty. This change allows personal relationships to be reinterpreted as environments that support self-acceptance without being constrained by social norms.

In this situation, communication becomes an effective tool for empowerment. Plus-sized people experience a mental change where they see open communication with partners as crucial. Destigmatizing discussions about preferences, boundaries, and desires fosters a supportive and understanding environment. This change encourages a more transparent and conversational approach to intimacy by challenging the stigma around talking about body size.

3. Prioritizing Comfort and Pleasure: One of the most important strategies for navigating happiness in close relationships is to adopt a mentality that puts comfort and pleasure ahead of social expectations. Plus-sized people learn to emphasize the delight and fulfillment that come from intimate relationships rather than conforming to conventional assumptions about their bodies. People start to prioritize their pleasure and realize that their contentment is independent of their ability to live up to social norms.

Furthermore, comfort becomes the guiding factor when it comes to personal settings. Mindset adjustments support plus-sized people in selecting activities and positions that suit their interests and level of comfort, creating a setting that makes both partners feel comfortable. This change casts doubt on the idea that some body types are better suited for intimate activities, encouraging a positive and satisfying sexual experience.

4. Empowering Self-Image in Sexual Expression: Among other important mental shifts, this one focuses on plus-sized people's ability to express themselves sexually. This change confirms that body size has no bearing on one's level of sexual confidence. Plus-sized people understand that being confident in the bedroom is a right, not a privilege, and that they should be able to express their sexuality with confidence.

A fundamental part of this mentality shift is the exploration and acceptance of various types of sexual expression. Plus-sized people defy social norms and give themselves permission to partake in fulfilling and pleasurable activities. This change encourages a more accepting perspective on sexual expression by highlighting the fact that pleasure in close relationships is not dependent on a specific bodily type or range of activities.

The way plus-sized people achieve happiness when it comes to sex and being overweight is greatly impacted by mental adjustments. It is clear how embracing a body-positive perspective, eradicating social stigmas, encouraging open communication, putting comfort and pleasure first, and empowering oneself in sexual expression can improve one's life. These changes question established conventions, encourage diversity, and acknowledge that happiness in close relationships is a personal and varied experience. Plus-sized people set out on a path to self-acceptance, confidence, and true happiness in their personal lives by implementing these mental changes. The narrative surrounding plus-sized people becomes more inclusive and gratifying when it is realized that intimate bliss is not limited to specific body types but can be attained via self-love and positive thought modifications.

3. Positive Self-Talk

In the path of plus-sized people exploring happiness in the context of sex and society perceptions of being overweight, positive self-talk emerges as a powerful force of empowerment. A transformative experience can be facilitated by altering internal narratives, developing self-compassion, reaffirming limits and desires, and boosting resilience and confidence through encouraging self-talk. This internal conversation turns into a source of strength, helping people to accept their individuality, communicate their desires honestly, and successfully negotiate close relationships.

Positive affirmations that highlight one's own qualities and strengths help cultivate a more resilient outlook. People are directed toward constructive self-reflection rather than focusing on their alleged flaws. This entails taking lessons from past mistakes, recognizing personal development, and reinterpreting obstacles as chances for improvement.

The transforming potential of positive self-talk in promoting resilience, self-empowerment, and a positive self-perception loop is looked at in the following paragraphs. These are vital components in the pursuit of happiness for people who must contend with societal judgments regarding their body size.

Changing Internal Narratives: For plus-sized people, positive self-talk starts a significant internal narrative transformation. In terms of sex and how society views being overweight, it entails purposefully refuting and contesting the myths that have been molded by cultural standards. People have a conversation that celebrates their individuality rather than internalizing negative stereotypes, which helps them develop a positive self-perception that is resistant to criticism from others.

Sexual relationships are particularly affected by this change in internal narratives. Positive self-talk turns into a tool for changing the way people think about their wants, bodies, and worth. It disproves the idea that physical attractiveness is limited to particular body types, opening the door for a welcoming and affirming narrative that supports pursuing happiness on one's own terms.

Building Self-Compassion: The foundation of positive self-talk is the development of self-compassion, which is a potent defense against expectations and judgments from society. Positive self-talk teaches plus-sized people to be kind and understanding to themselves in their quest of happiness. This entails admitting that everyone is deserving of love, happiness, and fulfillment regardless of their physical appearance.

Cultivating self-compassion becomes crucial when it comes to sex. People who use positive self-talk are more likely to accept and enjoy their bodies and realize that their value is independent of their ability to live up to social norms. This change in perspective creates a climate of self-affirmation where people may confidently negotiate personal situations without feeling constrained by social norms.

Affirming Limits and Wants: In close relationships, positive self-talk can be a useful technique for establishing limits and confirming wants. Due to the pressures from society, plus-sized people learn how to speak to themselves in a way that affirms their needs and establishes limits. This change helps to create an environment in which people feel free to voice their needs without sacrificing their sense of value.

A crucial component of dealing with happiness in the context of sex is using positive self-talk to validate boundaries and wants. It makes it possible for people to speak honestly with their relationships, which promotes understanding and creates an atmosphere in which both can feel happy and fulfilled. This change promotes authenticity in close relationships and contests the idea that people who identify as plus-sized should live up to stereotypes.

Building Resilience and Confidence: For plus-sized people, positive self-talk is essential to fostering resilience and confidence. People engage in an internal debate that validates their worth and ability in the face of society judgments and prejudices. This change helps people become more resilient by enabling them to face obstacles head-on and with confidence.

Building resilience and confidence through constructive self-talk can have a transforming effect on sex. It gives people the freedom to approach private moments without the limitations of social conventions and with a good self-image. This change in perspective creates a space where people who identify as plus-sized can confidently explore their sexuality and embrace a variety of expressions without worrying about being judged.

Positive self-talk transforms into a revolutionary act of self-love and self-empowerment in the pursuit of happiness. It refutes external narratives that attempt to define value on the basis of body size and celebrates the intrinsic worth and deservingness of plus-sized people. People create a route to happiness through positive self-talk that is based on self-love, authenticity, and the unshakeable conviction that every body, whatever of size, is worthy of happiness and fulfillment.

4. Setting Personal Boundaries: Developing assertiveness skills is a component of resilience building. People acquire the ability to clearly define and express their personal boundaries, which helps them to deal with social demands without sacrificing their morals or wellbeing. Being able to say 'no' when it's necessary helps you build confidence. This gives people the ability to put their needs first and resist giving in to pressure from outside sources that might not be consistent with who they really are.

5. Self-Compassion Practices: Developing self-compassion is a necessary skill for overcoming social pressures. By teaching themselves to be as understanding and kind to themselves as they would be to a friend, people create a loving and encouraging internal conversation. People are urged to regard setbacks as chances for personal development rather than as failures. This change in perspective makes failures more

manageable by turning them into opportunities for growth and development.

6. Seeking Support Networks: People who are developing resilience and self-confidence actively look for and take care of helpful relationships. These networks bolster people's resilience in the face of social pressures by offering support, empathy, and a feeling of community. In support networks, candid communication entails disclosing obstacles and experiences. People feel more empowered as a group as a result of realizing they are not alone in their quest to develop resilience.

7. Skill Development and Personal Growth: A dedication to lifelong learning is entwined with the development of confidence. People are encouraged to explore their interests, pick up new skills, and take part in activities that advance their professional and personal development. Accepting difficulties is a key component of resilience. People come to understand that conquering challenges, despite the discomfort involved, enhances

their resilience and ability to adjust to external influences.

8. Mindfulness and Self-Care: Developing resilience and self-confidence can be facilitated by practicing mindfulness. People can react to social pressure in a purposeful and genuine way when they are self-aware and live in the present. Making self-care a priority helps maintain resilience. Good sleep habits, a balanced diet, and enjoyable hobbies all support a solid base for developing and sustaining self-confidence.

2. Exploring Paths for Self-Discovery and Accepting Personal Satisfaction Despite External Evaluations

In the search for happiness, especially for plus-sized people facing social criticism, it can be a life-changing experience to pursue self-improvement paths. Here, we will examine the value of accepting personal fulfillment above and beyond criticism from others, negotiating the challenges of self-discovery, and creating a happy path apart from society norms.

Recognizing the Effect of Outside Opinions: Prior to exploring paths of self-discovery, it is critical to recognize how outside opinions affect people who identify as plus-sized. Unrealistic beauty standards are frequently imposed by society, which feeds prejudices and creates an atmosphere in which people may feel alienated or condemned because of their body size. The first step to handling happiness with resilience and authenticity is realizing this outside influence.

External opinions have a significant impact on people in the complex content of the human experience, and for those who identify as plus-sized, treading the emotional terrain molded by society beliefs can be a challenging path. Gaining insight into how outside opinions affect plus-sized people requires a careful examination of the complex emotional terrain they must traverse. External assessments have a lasting impact on people, informing social relationships, body image, and self-esteem, among other psychological effects. Understanding the subtle emotional aspects is essential for developing cultures that celebrate variety, encourage self-acceptance, and support plus-sized people as they pursue pleasure and fulfillment. It also lays the groundwork for developing empathy.

Let's look deeply into the complex effects of outside opinions on those who identify as plus-sized, illuminating the subtle emotional dynamics and difficulties that come when one's expectations are met.

Self-Esteem and Body Image: One of the most important aspects of the emotional environment for plus-sized people is the influence of outside judgments on self-esteem and body image. Narrow beauty standards are frequently imposed by society, and people who do not fit it may find their self-esteem damaged. Negative body image is a result of external evaluations that weaken one's sense of self-worth and encourage feelings of inadequacy.

The ongoing scrutiny and social demands placed on plus-sized people might make them feel like they don't measure up.

Relationships, professional goals, and general well-being are all impacted by this influence on body image and self-esteem. Comprehending this psychological cost is essential for managing the journey towards resilience and self-acceptance.

Psychological Repercussions: The mental health of plus-sized people can be negatively impacted by a variety of psychological effects that can arise from external evaluations. Anxiety, despair, and other mental health issues might result from society pressure to meet particular bodily ideals. Internalizing unfavorable assessments can start a self-doubt loop that makes people feel more emotionally burdened.

Additionally, being constantly exposed to social expectations can increase feelings of guilt or shame, which exacerbates the psychological difficulties that plus-sized people encounter. Comprehending the psychological ramifications of external judgments is crucial in addressing their wider influence and putting methods to support mental health and well-being into action.

Social Communication and Connections:
For plus-sized people, outside opinions have an impact on relationships and social interactions as well. Social disengagement or reluctance to make new friends may result from a fear of being judged or rejected due to one's body size. This effect also extends to romantic relationships, where the pursuit of meaningful connections may be hampered and confidence affected by society beauty standards.

External evaluations have a variety of emotional effects on social relationships. People who are plus-sized may have increased self-consciousness in public settings, which can hinder their ability to interact with people in a genuine way. In order to develop empathy and create situations that support inclusivity and acceptance, it is imperative to understand these relationships.

Adaptive Strategies and Resilience:
Examining coping strategies and resilience is necessary to comprehend the effects of outside opinions. In order to deal with

societal expectations, plus-sized people frequently create coping mechanisms. These could include building an effective support system or strengthening their inner fortitude. Understanding these coping strategies is essential to appreciating the resilience and ingenuity of people who must deal with criticism from others.

In order to lessen the emotional burden of societal perceptions, resilience becomes crucial. Gaining knowledge about how plus-sized people overcome obstacles, develop coping strategies, and foster resilience might help people strengthen their defenses against the psychological effects of criticism from others.

1. Embracing Self-Discovery: An Empowering Journey for Individuals Who Identify as Plus-Sized

For plus-sized people, accepting self-discovery becomes a transforming journey in the complex fabric of human growth. For plus-sized people, accepting self-discovery becomes a life-changing journey that goes beyond the limitations of other people's perceptions. People set out on a path that honors authenticity and resilience by developing self-awareness, investigating interests and hobbies, emotional intelligence, and personal beliefs.

This is a journey not just about self-discovery, but also about accepting and honoring each and every aspect of who you are. When it comes to self-discovery, plus-sized people have the fortitude to defy social norms, rewrite history, and pursue happiness on their own terms. It is a path of self-love, empowerment, and the unshakeable conviction that each and every person, regardless of size, has a special essence that should be honored.

We'll explore the journey's deep relevance and how self-discovery can be a potent driver for resilience, authenticity, and pursuing happiness outside of social norms.

1. The Formation of Self-Awareness: The path of accepting self-discovery begins with developing self-awareness. People who are plus-sized take a deep look inside themselves, exploring the depths of their feelings, ideas, and goals. By developing self-awareness, people can expose the true essence of who they are by removing social pressures and outside opinions.

Being self-aware helps plus-sized people recognize their values, goals, and assets. It becomes a guiding light. This fundamental facet of self-discovery equips people to live authentically and clearly, setting the stage for a path towards true happiness.

2. Examining Hobbies and Interests: An important step in accepting self-discovery is looking into interests and pastimes. People who identify as plus-sized proactively pursue pursuits that offer them happiness,

contentment, and a feeling of direction. Pursuing interests that align with one's passions promotes a connection to one's true self, surpassing social norms and honoring individual differences.

Indulging in interests and hobbies, be it in the arts, sports, literature, or any other field, serves as a conduit for plus-sized people to uncover aspects of themselves that go beyond what is seen from the outside. In addition to fostering personal development, this exploratory trip provides a source of resilience against social expectations.

3. Develop Emotional Intelligence:
Developing emotional intelligence is essential to navigating the terrain of self-discovery. Plus-sized people know how important it is to comprehend and properly control their emotions. When it comes to navigating the challenges of self-acceptance and resiliency in the face of criticism from others, emotional intelligence serves as a compass.

People who have developed their emotional intelligence are more equipped to deal with society's expectations in a genuine and graceful manner. The process of self-exploration is closely linked to the development of emotional resilience, which empowers persons who identify as plus-sized to effectively manage obstacles, establish strong connections, and maintain a positive self-perception.

4. Understanding Personal Values: Accepting self-discovery involves investigating one's own values, the fundamental ideas that shape one's identity and feeling of purpose. Those who identify as plus-sized set out to comprehend and conform to these ideals, realizing that living in accordance with one's core convictions is the path to authenticity.

Knowing one's own values turns into a compass that directs actions and influences decisions made in life. This part of self-discovery gives plus-sized people the tools they need to negotiate society expectations while being true to who they are, which promotes a sense of fulfillment based on moral integrity.

2. Accepting Self-fulfillment Independent of Opinions from Others

For plus-sized people, the path of embracing personal fulfillment beyond criticism from others represents a significant release. For plus-sized people, embracing personal fulfillment above and beyond criticism from others is a liberating path. People redefine happiness on their own terms and reclaim their story by focusing on intrinsic value, developing a good body image, creating personal objectives, recognizing accomplishments, and fostering genuine connections.

This trip is a celebration of genuineness, tenacity, and the unshakable conviction that cultural norm compliance does not define one's level of personal fulfillment. It is an empowering journey that frees plus-sized people from the limitations of other people's perceptions, enabling them to live authentically, joyfully, and with a deep sense of fulfillment. Seeking how this journey might lead to authenticity, fortitude, and the pursuit of happiness free from social constraints, let's explore its transforming potential.

Turning the Lens to Internal Value: A fundamental change of perspective from societal expectations to intrinsic value is necessary as a first step toward accepting personal fulfillment beyond the opinions of others. People who identify as plus-sized understand how important it is to accept oneself regardless of how others may see you. This change becomes a statement that human fulfillment is an intrinsic right and is not dependent on meeting preconceived notions of beauty.

Acknowledging intrinsic value sets people on a path toward self-acceptance and love. This change promotes a good self-image, empowering plus-sized people to embrace their special attributes and understand that happiness is an internal process that is unaffected by opinions from others.

Creating a Positive Body Image: Developing a positive body image is essential to embracing personal fulfillment. Although society frequently sets unattainable beauty standards, this journey inspires plus-sized people to defy these expectations. It's about appreciating the body for what it is, flaws and all, and acknowledging that beauty comes in many forms.

A radical act of self-love is developing a positive body image. Plus-sized people develop a sense of pride and confidence by learning to see their bodies as allies rather than enemies. This part of the journey helps to create an environment in which people may live their lives free from the burden of social criticism and with a good self-image.

Setting Personal Objectives and Honoring Successes: Setting goals that are in line with one's values and aspirations is a necessary step toward embracing personal fulfillment. Plus-sized people set their own standards for success in their relationships, careers, and personal development. This part of the trip is about taking back control of one's life and writing one's own story.

Achieving personal goals becomes a source of fulfillment for the individual as well as a sign of accomplishment. It's an acknowledgment that every success, regardless of what society may expect, is a reflection of the fortitude and resiliency of the person. This journey promotes a positive view on life by encouraging the celebration of accomplishments.

Building Genuine Relationships: The path to personal fulfillment includes developing sincere relationships with both oneself and other people. People who identify as plus-sized understand how important it is to be around people who value and celebrate who they are. This entails cultivating relationships based on acceptance, tolerance, and respect for one another.

Building genuine relationships is a crucial part of achieving personal contentment. The idea is to establish a structure of support that empowers and encourages people, thereby reaffirming the notion that true connections that transcend criticism from others are the source of happiness.

For plus-sized people, finding happiness requires a two-pronged approach: exploring paths to self-awareness and accepting personal fulfillment independent of opinions from others. By developing their self-awareness, pursuing their hobbies, and strengthening their emotional intelligence, people can set out on a self-discovery path that serves as the cornerstone of true pleasure.

Building a healthy body image, appreciating personal accomplishments, and moving the emphasis from outside criticism to intrinsic worth are all part of embracing personal fulfillment. By empowering plus-sized people to determine their own happiness, this comprehensive approach promotes self-love, resilience, and a sense of fulfillment that goes beyond social norms. Regardless of body type, everyone can choose a path that is in line with their true self when it comes to self-actualization and happiness.

Chapter Three: Exploring Best Sex Positions for Plus-Size Individuals

The search for a happy and satisfied sexual life is a common goal in the world of personal relationships. Knowing and experimenting with the ideal sex positions becomes essential to fostering an inclusive and joyful environment for plus-sized people. Discovering the ideal sex positions for people of plus size involves a complex journey that combines variety, comfort, and closeness. It's a journey that goes beyond preconceptions, putting the creation of inclusive and enjoyable experiences and celebrating a variety of body types first.

This chapter digs into the exploration of plus-size-friendly sex positions, highlighting coziness, closeness, and the appreciation of various body shapes.

Positions Stressing Comfort and Accessibility: When it comes to comfort and accessibility, there are several sex positions that are particularly good for those who are plus-sized. An ageless classic, spooning provides a comfortable environment with little physical exertion. Another option is the modified missionary position, which relieves joint pressure while offering support. This category is completed by side-to-side posture, which promotes a laid-back and intimate atmosphere.

These roles emphasize plus-size people's physical health, making comfort and ease of movement the main priorities. By doing this, they foster an atmosphere that is favorable to interaction, communication, and the general enjoyment of private times.

Positions that Promote Intimacy and Connection: The foundation of a fulfilling sexual encounter is intimacy and connection. It becomes clear that choosing to be face-to-face is a meaningful decision since it promotes intense feelings of connection, emotional intimacy, and eye contact. Along with intimacy, seated positions like straddling or sitting on a partner's lap also give you a sensation of control over the encounter.

Positions that include erotic massage are included in this category, enhancing the personal experience by adding sensuous touch and heightened sensations. These positions enhance the overall closeness of the experience by placing a higher priority on sensory pleasure and emotional connection.

Positions that Encourage Variety and Exploration: A healthy and fulfilling sexual life greatly benefits from variety and exploration. Thoughtfully modified for plus-size people, doggie style variants provide comfort and versatility. These positions ensure a comfortable and supportive experience while accommodating varying angles and depths with the use of cushions or adjustments.

Plus-size people have the opportunity to take charge and adjust the pacing to suit their comfort levels by adopting the cowgirl and reverse cowgirl positions. By introducing a firm platform, standing or leaning adds a variation element that lets partners try out various depths and angles.

Here, communication, flexibility, and a shared knowledge of preferences are essential. Partners can co-create a sexual experience that celebrates diversity and increases the joy, fulfillment, and connection of intimate times by creating an atmosphere that acknowledges the special requirements and comfort levels of plus-size people. Intimacy can be richer and more rewarding when inclusivity and celebrating individuality become the guiding principles in the search of sexual happiness.

Beyond just physical mechanics, a review of the ideal sex positions for plus-size people also includes debunking myths and stereotypes that have frequently surrounded the private lives of people with a variety of body types.

This part explores the significance of questioning stereotypes, advocating for diversity, and cultivating a more accurate understanding of sex for those who identify as plus-size.

1. Rid yourself of the Myths and Stereotypes About Sex for People of Plus Size

The idea that physical appearance and body size are correlated is one widespread myth. In order to debunk this stereotype, one must question the idea that certain physical shapes are preferable to others. Plus-size people can be proud of their distinctive features, and beauty is not limited by social conventions.

One of the biggest obstacles that plus-size people have in the world of personal relationships is the widespread impact of body image prejudices. It is a transforming endeavor to challenge body image norms, as doing so goes beyond changing cultural opinions. It involves redefining beauty and desire for plus-size individuals on both a personal and a community level. Through debunking the concept of a monolithic ideal, honoring individuality, advocating genuine portrayal, and fostering self-esteem, society can progress toward a more comprehensive and validating definition of beauty—one that acknowledges and appreciates the elegance innate in variety. In addition to helping plus-size people, this change also advances a larger cultural movement that values and celebrates the diverse range of human bodies.

In the following paragraphs, we'll look at how critical it is to confront these prejudices, demolish unattainable beauty standards, and promote a more accepting definition of attractiveness and desire for people of different body shapes.

Comprehending Stereotypes About Body Image:

Stereotypes about body image frequently depict a narrow variety of body types as desirable, perpetuating unattainable and constrictive ideals of beauty. These misconceptions about plus-size people might cause them to feel inadequate, self-conscious, and like they don't live up to society expectations. In the area of intimacy, it is imperative to challenge these preconceptions in order to foster self-acceptance and create a more accepting atmosphere for people who identify as plus-size.

1. Busting the Stupid Idea of a Singular Ideal: Dispelling the assumption that there is a single ideal of beauty is the first step towards combating misconceptions about body image. Attractiveness is a personal opinion, and beauty comes in many forms. Like everyone else, plus-size people have certain characteristics that draw others to them. Society can overcome the constraints imposed by preconceptions and appreciate the richness of diversity in physical appearance by adopting a more inclusive definition of beauty.

2. Honoring Distinctiveness and Special Qualities: In order to challenge negative stereotypes about body image, plus-size people must embrace their individuality and celebrate what makes them special. Everybody's body reveals something about their experiences, resiliency, and individuality. Through prioritizing the celebration of unique attributes over

uniformity, society can cultivate a more optimistic and tolerant outlook towards a varied range of body types.

3. Encouragement of Realistic Representation: Advertising and the media have a big influence on how society views beauty. In order to dispel misconceptions about body image, authentic representations of a range of body types must be encouraged in popular media. This involves presenting plus-size people in a variety of settings, such as close relationships, in order to subvert the constrictive stereotypes that are upheld by traditional representations.

4. Promoting Acceptance and Self-Love: Promoting self-love and acceptance is a crucial part of combating misconceptions surrounding body image on a personal level. Plus-size people can start the process of accepting their bodies and realizing that attractiveness isn't limited to a particular size or shape. Building a positive self-image and resisting outside criticism are made possible by practicing self-love.

Busting Performance Myths

It's a common misperception that people who are plus-sized may have difficulties when it comes to their sexual performance. Realizing that body size has no bearing on sexual enjoyment is the first step in busting this misconception. A satisfying sex experience involves open communication, trust, and exploring positions that are optimized for comfort and pleasure.

Myths about plus-size people's sexual performance add to preconceived notions that could undermine their self-worth and enjoyment of close relationships. It's critical to address performance myths for plus-size people in order to build sexual confidence, demolish irrational expectations, and cultivate a more true perception of pleasure and capacity. By dispelling myths, emphasizing communication and connection, investigating flexible positions, encouraging sexual confidence, and raising consciousness, society can help to foster a society where close relationships are valued in all of its varied forms.

This change benefits plus-size people as well as improving the conversation about sexuality in general by highlighting the fact that people of all body types may find contentment and joy.

Let's look at the significance of dispelling these performance myths, highlighting the truth that physical appearance has no bearing on one's level of sexual happiness, and advocating for a more realistic conception of pleasure and competence.

1. Dispelling Myths About Performance: The perception that plus-size people may have difficulties with sexual performance is frequently reinforced by performance stereotypes. These false beliefs have the potential to cause worry, self-doubt, and communication problems in relationships. Dispelling these myths requires acknowledging that, rather than being primarily determined by physical appearance, sexual fulfillment is a complex experience characterized by mutual consent, communication, and emotional connection.

2. Putting Connection and Communication First: Dispelling performance misconceptions emphasizes how important emotional ties and communication are in close relationships. Like everyone else, plus-size people do best in relationships when partners value honest communication, clearly state wants and boundaries, and build a foundation of trust. An environment that prioritizes communication above irrational expectations makes for a more fulfilling and healthful sexual experience.

3. Exploring Comfort-Core Positions: Exploring sex positions that are comfortable is one useful strategy for busting performance myths. Understanding that bodies vary widely in size and shape, couples might try different positions to suit the particular demands and preferences of plus-size people in terms of their physical appearance. This investigation places a strong emphasis on flexibility, reciprocal fulfillment, and realizing that there are several ways to experience sexual pleasure.

4. Promoting Sexual Confidence and Autonomy: In order to dispel performance clichés, plus-size people must be encouraged to feel confident and independent in their sexuality. Instead of being dependent on meeting rigid social norms, confidence in the bedroom is based on communication, self-acceptance, and a shared dedication to enjoyment and contentment. Encouraging a setting in which people feel free to voice their wants and actively participate in their sexual encounters enhances their general sense of contentment and well-being.

5. Raising Awareness and Educating: Dispelling performance misconceptions necessitates a larger social education and awareness campaign. It is crucial to spread accurate knowledge about sexual health, capacities, and the range of intimate encounters. By dispelling misconceptions, lowering stigma, and promoting a more accepting and compassionate viewpoint on sexual fulfillment for plus-size people, this education helps.

Encouraging Communication and Consent

Another misconception is that talking about sex-related desires or worries could make plus-size people feel awkward. Breaking down this myth highlights how crucial it is to have honest conversations and get consent. Establishing a relationship based on communication and trust allows both partners to freely express their boundaries and desires.

Encouraging consent and communication is essential to building happy, healthy intimate relationships, especially for plus-size people who might encounter extra difficulties because of cultural prejudices. Encouraging consent and communication is essential for fostering healthy intimate relationships as well as a means of subverting prejudices and social standards that may negatively affect people of plus-size. Through recognizing the value of communication, establishing safe spaces for candid conversations, instituting consistent consent procedures, teaching affirmative consent, and using communication to dispel stereotypes, society can help to create an atmosphere in which people of all body types feel respected, empowered, and free to engage in intimate relationships in an authentic way. Plus-size people benefit from this cultural change toward open communication and permission, which also strengthens relationships by highlighting the need for respect and mutual understanding as necessary components of satisfying interpersonal relationships.

We will examine how important it is to have open lines of communication and consent in order to foster an atmosphere that values respect, understanding, and the empowerment of people with all different types of bodies.

1. Recognizing the Value of Communication
The foundation of any healthy relationship, even close ones, is effective communication. Creating an environment where partners feel at ease talking about needs, boundaries, and concerns is important for plus-sized people. This understanding necessitates a departure

from cultural traditions that could obstruct candid communication and create a more encouraging and welcoming atmosphere.

2. Establishing Secure Environments for Free Speech:.Establishing secure areas for candid discussion is part of fostering communication. It should be acceptable for partners to communicate their wants, preferences, and doubts without worrying about being judged. Being able to manage intimate relationships with confidence and sincerity is especially important for plus-size individuals who may have faced prejudice or stereotypes from society.

3. Creating Consistent Consent Procedures: Consent is a mutually enthusiastic and continuing agreement between all parties. It is an essential component of civilized and consenting small talk. Encouraging partners to articulate and uphold their boundaries as well as actively seek affirmative agreement at every level of closeness are all important aspects of promoting consistent consent practices.

4. Teaching About Positive Consent: People need to be educated about affirmative consent as a group in order to encourage communication and consent. The concept of affirmative consent highlights the significance of willing and enthusiastic consent during personal relationships. This knowledge is essential for dispelling myths and enabling plus-size people to openly express their boundaries and wants.

5. Handling Stereotypes With Honest Conversation: When negotiating societal prejudices, communication becomes an extremely useful weapon. Partners can address preconceived beliefs, debunk falsehoods, and promote understanding through open communication. Couples can create an environment that is supportive of various body shapes and resistant to outside criticism by talking about expectations and working through possible difficulties jointly.

Recognizing Diverse Desires
The oversimplification of plus-size people's goals is a prevalent stereotype. Realizing the variety of desires within this group is

essential to dispelling this fallacy. As is the case with people of any size, preferences are very diverse. A more comprehensive and sophisticated viewpoint is facilitated by comprehending and recognizing these varied aspirations.

Sexual relationship diversity must start with acknowledging different desires, especially for plus-size people who could be negatively impacted by prejudices in society. Promoting tolerance and understanding in intimate relationships, particularly for plus-sized people, requires acknowledging the diversity of aspirations.

Society may help create a more accepting and affirming environment by challenging stereotypes, valuing human complexity, embracing personal autonomy, promoting inclusive sexual education, and fostering open communication between partners. This cultural change emphasizes that wants are diverse, complicated, and individually personal, regardless of body size, which benefits plus-size people as well as enriching the larger conversation on human sexuality.

We will explore how important it is to acknowledge and celebrate the variety of wants found within this diverse group, bust myths, and advance the idea that enjoyment is personal to each person, regardless of size.

1. Debunking Stupid Assumptions: The oversimplification of plus-size people's desires is one common issue. The understanding of this group's varied and complex desires is frequently hampered by stereotypes. Breaking down stereotypes means acknowledging that people with different body types have distinct tastes, fantasies, and desires that don't fit into one story.

2. Appreciating Personal Complexity: Recognizing varied aspirations means appreciating the unique complexity of every person's personal choices. This is a celebration that goes beyond the material and includes relational, psychological, and emotional factors. Society may break free from constrictive assumptions and acknowledge that pleasure is as varied as

the people who experience it by recognizing the complexity of desires.

3. Accepting Individual Agency: People have the agency to explore and truly express their aspirations, regardless of their body size. Embracing personal agency means fostering an atmosphere in which people who identify as plus-size feel free to express their needs and desires honestly. This change encourages a society that respects individuality and recognizes that people are the experts on their own wishes.

4. Encouraging Comprehensive Sexual Education: To acknowledge the diversity of desires, one must be dedicated to advancing inclusive sexual education. The main goals of educational initiatives should be to debunk misconceptions, confront stereotypes, and give truthful information about the variety of wants that plus-size people can have. A more knowledgeable and compassionate society that embraces the diversity of human sexuality is fostered by this inclusive approach.

5. Promoting Free and Honest
Communication Between Partners:
Recognizing different desires in close
partnerships requires open communication.
It should be easy for partners to talk about
preferences, investigate imaginations, and
work through desires in tandem. Couples can
strengthen their bonds and establish
environments where both partners feel
appreciated and understood without bias or
presumptions about one another's bodies by
encouraging an open culture.

Beyond physicality, the ideal sex positions for
plus-size people are explored to challenge
assumptions and dispel myths. We work to
create a more accurate and inclusive view of
sex for people with a variety of body types
by addressing prejudices surrounding body
image, dispelling myths about performance,
encouraging communication and consent,
and recognizing the range of wants.

This change in viewpoint not only benefits
plus-size people's confidence and general
well-being, but it also advances the idea that
sexual fulfillment is varied, complex, and

unrestricted by social conventions. Eliminating stereotypes based on personal relationships is essential to fostering an accepting and affirming atmosphere where everyone may enjoy themselves, connect with others, and find fulfillment without having to bear the burden of false belie

2. An All-Inclusive Guide to Various Comfortable and Enjoyable Sexual Positions for Various Body Shapes

Developing an extensive manual on various, cozy, and enjoyable sexual poses for various body shapes is a worthwhile project to promote diversity and improve personal relationships. The development of a thorough manual on various, enjoyable, and pleasant sex positions for various body shapes is a step in the direction of encouraging a more affirming and inclusive perspective on close partnerships. Through highlighting flexibility, placing a premium on comfort, and acknowledging the range of personal preferences, this following paragraphs seeks to facilitate a cultural transformation that embraces the individuality and beauty of every body. In the end, the objective is to offer a tool that encourages contentment, happiness, and connection for people of all shapes and sizes, supporting a more inclusive perspective of sexual experience.

In order to accommodate a wide variety of body types, this guide attempts to offer a selection of positions that put comfort, versatility, and enjoyment first.

Recognizing the Value of Diversity

Understanding that different people have different bodies is essential to creating a guide that works for a wide range of people. This knowledge challenges preconceptions and celebrates the individuality of every person's body, encouraging an inclusive perspective on close connections.

For overweight people, diversity in sex is crucial for many reasons beyond just physical ones. It encompasses a wide range of wants, experiences, and the appreciation of special connections.

Recognizing the significance of variety in sexual experiences for overweight people is a thorough understanding of every aspect that goes into creating a happy and meaningful intimate life. Society may help bring about a cultural shift that celebrates the diversity of human sexuality by opposing stigmatization, recognizing a range of wants, supporting inclusive representation, enabling open communication, and building mutual respect.

This change is beneficial to overweight people as well as the larger conversation about intimacy since it highlights the fact that all people, regardless of size, should feel fulfilled, connected, and happy in their personal relationships.

Let's explore the complex meaning of accepting variety in the personal lives of overweight people, emphasizing representation, inclusivity, and fostering an atmosphere that values the range of human sexuality.

1. Taking On Body Shaming and Stigmatization: Diversity in sexual relationships for people who are overweight is essential to combating body shaming and stigma that are pervasive in society norms. By accepting a wide variety of body shapes, we can break down negative preconceptions and create a space where people feel appreciated, welcomed, and unburdened by social norms. This fight against stigmatization fosters self-assurance and a good perception of one's physique.

2. Affirming Varied Desires and Preferences: Diversity acknowledges and affirms the varied desires and preferences within the overweight community. Recognizing that sexual pleasure is nuanced and personal, this understanding validates a spectrum of desires, creating a space where individuals can explore, express, and celebrate their unique preferences without judgment or limitation.

3. Fostering Inclusive Representation: In the context of diversity in sex, representation becomes a powerful tool. Fostering inclusive

representation in media, literature, and cultural narratives is crucial. Overweight individuals deserve to see themselves authentically represented in intimate scenarios, challenging stereotypes, and contributing to a more accurate portrayal of diverse relationships. This representation dismantles prejudices and fosters a sense of belonging.

4. Establishing an Open Communication Culture: Diversity in sexual orientation promotes the growth of an open communication culture. Open communication aids in addressing the special difficulties or worries that overweight people may have. People feel powerful, encouraged, and more competent navigating intimate relationships when partners can freely communicate wishes, boundaries, and concerns.

5. Encouraging Respect and Understanding Between People: Respect and understanding between partners are fostered by inclusive variety in the sexual sphere. It promotes an awareness of the distinctive viewpoints and experiences that every person brings to the

partnership. Respect for one another promotes closeness, emotional connection, and a shared discovery path that transcends physical characteristics.

1. Positions Focusing on Accessibility and Comfort in Overweight Persons' Sexual Pleasure

A universal human experience, sexual pleasure is one that should be celebrated and acknowledged for the variety of people's bodies and wants.

The celebration of various bodies and wants, as well as inclusivity and adaptability, are highlighted in this handbook to sexual enjoyment for overweight people. Through emphasizing ease, fostering emotional bonding, and allowing for exploration, people can design a sexual experience that celebrates their individuality and cultivates happiness. In order to make sure that the shared exploration of pleasure is a rewarding and meaningful experience for all parties involved, communication between couples is still crucial. Accepting these roles enables people to see past social norms and recognize the diversity and beauty present in every personal encounter.

The material here aims to give advice on sexual positions that are especially suitable for overweight people, with an emphasis on comfort, accessibility, and creating a pleasurable and fulfilling sexual experience.

A. Modified Missionary: Establishing Consistency and Closeness

For those who are overweight, the Modified Missionary position is made with stability and comfort in mind. The receiving partner offers a stable basis and relieves joint pressure by lying on their back with their knees slightly bent. The penetrating partner may choose to kneel or use self-support in the interim. In addition to providing for physical comfort, this arrangement encourages intimate physical and emotional bonding between partners. It offers a laid-back setting where both parties may converse honestly and take pleasure in an enjoyable experience without needless stress.

B. Spooning: Developing Closeness and Calm

The traditional and cozy position of spooning creates a special atmosphere for private moments. With the entering partner embracing the receiving partner from behind, both parties lie on their sides. By fostering a calm environment, this position reduces physical strain and facilitates a stronger emotional bond. This setup's simplicity makes it a great option for those who are overweight since it creates the feeling of comfort and intimacy that is necessary for a satisfying sexual encounter.

C. Side-to-Side: Versatility and Emotional Connection

Both partners lie on their sides, facing one another, in the Side-to-Side posture. This adaptable configuration accommodates a variety of motions and postures, meeting the specific needs of every person. In addition to being flexible, this role facilitates simple communication and promotes easy

communication and enhances the emotional connection between partners.
It provides a comfortable space for exploration and intimacy, emphasizing the importance of both physical and emotional well-being.

D. Variations of the Cowgirl/Reverse Cowgirl: Adaptable and Empowering

Reverse and Cowgirl Cowgirl versions provide the receiving partner more control over the intensity and tempo of the interaction. In these positions, the receiving partner is either facing away from or straddling the penetrating partner. This flexibility gives overweight people a sense of comfort and control in addition to meeting their own preferences. It places a strong emphasis on enjoying each other's company and provides a fun and encouraging environment for exploration.

E. Seated Positions: Adaptability and Face-to-Face Interaction

Seated positions provide flexibility and in-person engagement, with the receiving partner sitting on the penetrating partner's lap. This category contains several configurations and angles that encourage comfort and adaptation. These roles promote open communication and a shared discovery of pleasure in addition to accommodating a variety of tastes. Sitting positions offer support that makes the encounter more comfortable and enjoyable for both partners.

2. Positions That Promote Closeness and Intimacy

Sexual pleasure is a deep emotional bond between couples as well as a physical act. One intentional strategy for fostering emotional ties in relationships is the investigation of postures that promote closeness and connection. People can create a complete and emotionally enlivening experience by combining face-to-face exchanges, seated postures, sexual massage aspects, sensual spooning, and embracing positions with mutual gaze. This deliberate emphasis on emotional closeness improves the quality of intimate times overall and strengthens the bond between couples, creating a relationship that is nourished by both emotional and physical fulfillment.

Examining stances intended to promote closeness and connection, we can see how important they are for developing stronger emotional ties in partnerships.

A. Positions for Erotic Massage: Increasing Touch-Based Intimacy

One interesting technique to improve sexual pleasure is to add sensual massage positions to special occasions. Touch, whether it comes from one person giving or receiving, promotes emotional intimacy. By emphasizing tactile communication, these postures let couples explore and value one other's bodies, which deepens their connection and strengthens their sense of emotional closeness.

B. Sensual Spooning: Nurturing Affection and Physical Comfort

When one approaches spooning with an emphasis on emotional connection, the classic position takes on a sensual quality. A cocoon of warmth, both physically and emotionally, is formed when both couples are resting on their sides and one is holding the other from behind. This position promotes closeness between partners, creating a feeling of security and closeness that extends beyond the immediate act of intimacy.

C. Accepting Positions with Eye Contact: Strengthening Emotional Ties

Emotional ties are strengthened in positions that permit mutual gaze, in which partners can keep looking at each other the entire time. Maintaining eye contact while in sitting, face-to-face, or missionary positions adds another level of emotional intimacy. By encouraging openness and vulnerability, this deliberate gaze adds to a shared experience that goes beyond the tangible.

3. Positions that Promote Variety and Exploration

A universal human experience, sexual pleasure is one that should be celebrated and inclusive of people's varied bodies and wants. Exploration and variety-oriented positions specifically address the special needs and considerations of overweight people, promoting inclusivity and delight in close relationships. The focus is on diversity and ongoing exploration, whether via variants on the Doggy Style, empowering positions like Cowgirl, incorporating standing or leaning positions, investigating oral pleasure, or partaking in sensory play. In addition to celebrating the unique bodies of overweight people, this deliberate commitment to variety makes the experience of pleasure for both partners more vibrant, rewarding, and joyful.

We'll explore roles created especially to facilitate innovation and diversity in close relationships, with an emphasis on the particular requirements and issues faced by people who are overweight. People may build a fulfilling sexual experience that embraces their bodies and promotes joy, connection, and fulfillment by embracing diversity and purposeful exploration.

A. Doggy Styles Variation: Adapting for Ease and Discovery

Doggy Style modifications provide flexibility for comfort and exploration for overweight people. This is a flexible position that allows partners to adjust to each other's comfort levels while experimenting with angles, depth, and pacing. People can customize the experience to their liking by adding modifications like changing the angles or providing extra support like pillows. This flexibility not only meets the particular requirements of those who are overweight but also encourages exploration and variety, creating a dynamic and pleasurable encounter.

B. Cowgirl and Reverse Cowgirl: Adaptable and Empowering

Because of its high degree of customization and empowering quality, the Cowgirl and Reverse Cowgirl positions are particularly well-suited for overweight people. By giving the receiving partner authority over the duration and tempo of the interaction, these positions empower them. These positions are flexible enough to allow for experimenting with various angles, rhythms, and intensities. This personalization adds to a dynamic and unique experience by introducing a sense of exploration and variety in addition to satisfying individual tastes.

C. Adding Novelty and Excitement with Standing or Leaning Positions

For overweight people, positions that require standing or leaning against a firm surface offer a chance to spice up romantic relationships with a little excitement and originality. This can be very helpful since it brings about a transformation.

D. Diverse Oral Pleasure: Broadening the Sensual Investigation

For overweight people, oral pleasure postures provide a flexible way to increase their level of sensual exploration. By experimenting with different body positions, angles, and oral intimacy techniques, partners can find the most pleasurable position for themselves. Oral pleasure positions are versatile and promote reciprocal exploration and open communication, which leaves room for variety and exploration in this area of personal relationships.

E. Including Sensory Play: Appealing to a Variety of Senses

Beyond positions, adding sensory play becomes an important component in improving diversity and enjoyment for people who are overweight. This could entail using handcuffs, blindfolds, or other sensory-enhancing tools. Using all of the senses enhances the experience and lets lovers discover new aspects of closeness and pleasure. This intentional approach to variety fosters excitement, novelty, and ongoing exploration within intimate relationships.

Chapter Four: Cultivating a Fulfilling Sexual Life

Everyone wants to have a fulfilling sexual life, but those who struggle with being overweight may need to take special concerns into account.

A complete plan that incorporates self-acceptance, open communication, exploring comfortable postures, mindful sensuality, body positivity, and mutual enjoyment is necessary to help persons who are seeking pleasure while overweight lead successful sexual lives. By adhering to these guidelines, people can successfully negotiate the complexities of both personal fears and society expectations, creating a setting where close relationships not only provide fulfillment but also generate a greater sense of joy, connection, and fulfillment.

For individuals dealing with the challenges of body weight, this chapter emphasizes pleasure, communication, and a positive approach to intimacy as means of developing a meaningful sexual life.

Recognizing and Loving Your Body: Understanding and accepting one's body, regardless of weight, is the first step towards having a fulfilling sexual life. Recognizing each person's intrinsic beauty and deservingness is essential to overcoming both personal fears and society pressures. This positive self-image forms the basis for fulfilling interpersonal interactions.

Vulnerability and Communication: Maintaining an authentic sexual life requires open communication, especially for individuals overcoming the obstacles posed by being overweight. In a supportive setting where both parties can freely express their needs, talking to a partner about desires, boundaries, and insecurities can help. As partners' emotional bond grows and trust is established, vulnerability is transformed into a strength.

Examination of Cozy Positions:
Finding cozy and enjoyable poses that meet the special requirements of people who are overweight is crucial. Jobs like reverse cowgirl, modified missionary, spooning, and cowgirl and reverse cowgirl allow people to do what makes them feel good and comfortable. This deliberate exploration of postures encourages flexibility and puts the health of both partners first.

Conscious Sensuality and Emotion:
A fulfilling sexual life requires thoughtful sensuality that emphasizes the bond between intimate physical and emotional contact. A higher sense of enjoyment can be attained by employing the senses, expressing wants, and keeping the present moment in mind. Encouraging a deeper connection that goes beyond the physical creates a conducive atmosphere for fulfilling and meaningful sexual experiences.

Promoting Positive Body Image:
One of the most important things in helping overweight people have a satisfying sexual life is to promote body positivity. Embracing

different beauty standards and questioning society conventions are two ways to cultivate a healthy self-image. Individuals are more likely to participate in intimate interactions with joy and self-assurance when they feel good about their bodies and confident in them.

Incorporating Pleasure for Both Parties:
In order to have a successful sexual life, one must prioritize reciprocal pleasure and understand that both partners' satisfaction is necessary for a healthy and fulfilling sexual dynamic. Reinforcing the emotional tie between couples involves mutual exploration, understanding each other's desires, and establishing an environment where pleasure is shared.

1. Emphasizing Open Communication with Overweight People Seeking Pleasure in Sexual Activities

Open communication becomes essential for those traveling the complex and highly personal path to a healthy sexual life who also happen to be overweight. For overweight people looking to pursue sexual pleasure and have a satisfying sexual life, it is critical to emphasize open communication. This deliberate approach to talking fosters trust, navigates issues of body image, expresses emotional needs, establishes a secure space for discussion, and permits ongoing adaptation. Intimate relationships may be a journey toward mutual understanding, fulfillment, and joy when people cultivate connection through transparency.

We'll talk about the importance of putting an emphasis on open communication in sexual relationships and how it may improve understanding, trust, and ultimately the development of a fulfilling and fulfilling sexual life.

Developing Trust and Acknowledging Vulnerability: In a sexual relationship, developing trust and acknowledging vulnerability are the first steps towards open communication. Addressing issues, expressing desires, and talking about insecurities are all necessary for overweight people. When this openness is greeted with compassion and understanding, it builds a foundation of mutual trust. When partners feel comfortable expressing their wants and desires, this vulnerability turns into a source of strength.

Talking Openly About Wants and Boundaries: Being able to talk freely about wants and boundaries is essential to having a successful sexual life. Individuals who are overweight may have particular issues, therefore it's important for partners to be clear about expectations, comfort zones, and preferences in order to align their goals. In addition to making sure that both parties feel heard and understood, this proactive conversation prepares the ground for a more fulfilling and joyful sexual experience for both of them.

Handling Body Image Issues: For those who seek sex being overweight, discussing body image issues is an essential part of being open and honest. Open dialogue regarding one's own self-perception, societal pressures, and personal insecurities fosters a supportive and understanding environment for both partners. Couples can create an atmosphere that supports body positivity by discussing and resolving these issues jointly,

Expressing Emotional Needs: Intimacy goes beyond the physical, and open communication includes expressing emotional needs in a sexual relationship. Like everyone else, overweight people want validation and emotional connection. A more comprehensive and satisfying sexual life can be achieved through expressing affection, cultivating connection, and being honest about emotional needs.

Establishing a Safe Space for Conversation: Having a satisfying sexual life necessitates the creation of a safe space for conversation. Since people who are overweight may experience stigmatization or judgment from society, it is important to foster an atmosphere in which they feel free to express themselves. By exhibiting empathy, active listening, and a nonjudgmental demeanor, partners can actively support this and reinforce the idea that open communication is not just welcomed but encouraged.

Continuous Check-Ins and Adaptability: Maintaining an open line of communication in a sexual relationship necessitates ongoing check-ins and flexibility. Individuals' wants and desires change as they grow. A fulfilling sexual life is sustained over time by a continuous dialogue regarding changing circumstances, exploring new interests, and shifting preferences. These conversations should happen on a regular basis.

2. Promoting Mutual Trust, Understanding, and Emotional Bonds Between Couples

Building trust, understanding, and an emotional bond between partners becomes essential in the quest for an enjoyable sexual life for overweight people.
Encouraging emotional closeness, empathy, and trust between partners is a comprehensive strategy for helping overweight people have satisfying sexual relationships. Couples create an environment

that transcends simple satisfaction by fostering good body image, celebrating intimacy beyond the physical, acknowledging emotional needs, navigating sensitivity with empathy, comprehending unique considerations, and creating trust through openness. For those negotiating the difficulties of body weight, this deliberate attention on emotional connection leads to a deeper, more meaningful, and ultimately more rewarding sexual life.

Let's explore the importance of laying the groundwork for a relationship around these components and emphasize how they may transform a space to make intimacy both fulfilling and emotionally stimulating.

Developing Openness to Build Trust: Any successful sexual connection is built on trust. Building trust with overweight people starts with being upfront and honest in conversation. In order to communicate needs, worries, and boundaries without fear of criticism, partners must feel comfortable doing so. By being open and honest, it builds a foundation of trust that makes it possible for both parties to interact in private with mutual understanding and security.

Understanding Particular Concerns: Achieving a satisfying sexual life requires an understanding of the particular issues that overweight people may encounter. This entails being aware of social influences, dealing with any underlying fears, and initiating active dialogue around body image. Physical and emotional well-being are valued in an atmosphere created by partners who take the effort to comprehend and empathize with these factors.

Managing Sensitivity and Empathy: Managing sensitivity and empathy is essential for assisting overweight people in developing emotional connections. Couples should be sensitive to one another's emotions, aware of any potential sensitivities, and empathetic in their responses. A deeper connection is facilitated by this level of emotional intelligence, which fosters an environment in which both partners feel appreciated, understood, and emotionally supported.

Promoting a Positive Body Image: For overweight people, maintaining a positive body image is essential to developing a satisfying sexual life. Partners actively promote positive self-perception, which plays a vital part in this process. Acknowledgments, declarations of love, and compliments create a nurturing atmosphere that boosts self-esteem and confidence, improving the sex experience in general.

Honoring Intimacy Beyond Its Physical elements: Honoring intimacy beyond its physical elements is just as significant, even if physical closeness is an essential component. Sharing stories, giggling, and showing affection are all components of an emotional relationship. Actively connecting with each other in non-sexual moments strengthens a couple's bond beyond the bedroom and fosters an emotional contentment that improves the relationship as a whole.

Affirming Emotional Needs: For overweight people, fostering a fulfilling sexual life is mostly dependent on affirming their emotional needs. It is important for partners to actively communicate and fulfill each other's emotional needs, whether they are for companionship, assurance, or just spending time together. This encouragement strengthens the emotional bond that makes an intimate relationship more gratifying and satisfying.

3. Integrating Variety, Creativity, and the Significance of Intimacy

Embracing diverse activities, encouraging creativity in expression, celebrating the beauty of diverse bodies, incorporating sensory exploration, and experimenting with different environments all contribute to a deeply satisfying sexual experience. By placing a high priority on the multifaceted aspects of intimacy, couples can intentionally navigate the complexities of body weight and create a sexually fulfilling relationship.

We will look at how, for people, navigating the complexities of body weight, accepting diversity, encouraging creativity, and realizing the deeper meaning of intimacy contribute to a profoundly fulfilling sexual experience.

Accepting Diversities in Close Examining:
For overweight people to have a satisfying sexual life, variety is essential. Engaging in a variety of intimate pursuits, such as sensual massages and shared fantasies, enables partners to investigate many aspects of pleasure. The deliberate incorporation of diversity guarantees that sexual encounters sustain its dynamic, captivating nature, and customization to the distinct inclinations and comfort zones of each partner.

Encouraging Innovative Approaches to Sexual Expression:
Expressing oneself sexually creatively creates fresh opportunities and makes intimate interactions more satisfying overall. Trying various positions, providing role-play scenarios, or including sensual games are some inventive methods to connect

intimately with overweight people. This inventiveness fosters a shared feeling of amusement and exploration in the sexual connection in addition to bringing arousal.

Seeing Intimacy's Deeper Significance: A deeply fulfilling sexual experience is facilitated by an understanding of the underlying meaning of intimacy, which extends beyond physical pleasure. Like everyone else, overweight people want to feel important and connected emotionally. Emotionally intimate partners foster a climate of trust, understanding, and vulnerability that enriches the sexual experience in general.

Celebrating the Gift of Diverse Forms: Diversity includes celebrating a variety of body types. Regardless of social conventions, a healthy sexual life necessitates recognizing and celebrating each partner's distinct physical beauty. This celebration contributes to a more fulfilling and affirming sexual encounter by promoting body positivity and improving one's perception of attractiveness and desirability.

Including Sensory Investigation:
Intimate connections have an additional dimension of creativity and variation when sensory inquiry is incorporated. This can entail enhancing perceptions and producing a more immersive experience through the use of music, textures, or scents. By increasing one's awareness of one another's bodies through sensory exploration, a stronger bond is created and the enjoyment of private moments is intensified.

Playing Around in Various Environments:
The importance of closeness is increased when partners experiment with various settings for sex. A change of location, whether it be from your house, a weekend away, or even an impromptu outdoor activity, brings excitement and originality to your sexual relationship. This experience of exploring other environments adds to a feeling of fulfillment and adventure.

Chapter Five: Resources and Support for Overweight Individuals Seeking Sexual Fulfillment

The route towards sexual fulfillment is an intensely individualized one, influenced by personal experiences, goals, and obstacles. The availability of resources and a supportive network becomes essential in navigating this complex route for overweight individuals who are seeking sexual satisfaction. Lots of resources and a supportive network help overweight people on their path to sexual fulfillment. The availability of diverse resources enables people to confidently and resiliently navigate their unique path, whether through professional guidance, engagement with body-positive communities, access to educational resources, participation in inclusive workshops, healthcare consultations, supportive partnerships, or mental health support. People can develop a satisfying sexual life that not only celebrates their bodies and sexuality but also promotes overall well-being by embracing these resources and fostering a supportive network.

We will examine the wide array of available options and the significant influence of support networks on those who are embracing their sexual urges while managing the intricacies of their body weight.

Professional Advisers and Sexual Counselors: Expert counseling is a ray of hope for everyone seeking sexual fulfillment. With their extensive training in handling a wide range of sexual issues, sex therapists provide a secure environment for people figuring out the complexities of their wants, especially when it comes to body weight issues. Their nonjudgmental manner fosters an environment of open inquiry while offering customized counsel and techniques to develop a satisfying sexual life.

Body Positive Forums & Communities: One cannot emphasize the importance of community, particularly in the context of body positivity. Participating in online forums and body-positive networks offers a safe space for people to exchange stories, counsel, and support. These venues encourage a sense of belonging by showcasing the diversity of bodies. They develop into priceless places where people may find comfort and share wisdom, particularly those overcoming obstacles related to body weight.

Resources for Education on Body Positivity and Pleasure: Acquiring knowledge is an effective means of achieving sexual contentment. Books, articles, and internet sites are examples of educational tools that are essential in influencing attitudes toward pleasure and body acceptance. For people who are overweight, having access to information that celebrates different body types and promotes having a positive outlook about one's desires becomes empowering, challenging societal norms and fostering self-acceptance.

Classes and Workshops on Inclusive Sexuality: Enrolling in workshops and programs on inclusive sexuality is a proactive measure towards achieving personal empowerment. These expert-led seminars offer a secure and encouraging space for exploration on a variety of subjects, including body acceptance and communication techniques. These workshops become life-changing opportunities for overweight people to gain useful skills and insights that improve their sex lives.

Health Care Workers and Dietitians: Taking general health into account is a common component of a holistic approach to sexual wellness. Consulting with nutritionists and medical professionals enhances a person's overall health, which has a beneficial effect on their sexual health. A fulfilling sexual life is based on taking care of health issues, investigating dietary options, and preserving general wellbeing.

Friendly Partnerships and Honest Communication: One cannot overstate the importance of a helpful cooperation. An atmosphere of support is created in a relationship through open communication, where needs and fears are discussed and accepted. Relationships where empathy, good communication, and shared exploration are valued greatly increase the enjoyment of the sexual relationship as a whole.

Support for Mental Health: Sexual health and well-being are closely related. People who are overweight and may experience internalized stigmas and social pressures may find it helpful to seek out support groups or mental health specialists. Overcoming these obstacles cultivates an optimistic outlook that is favorable to accepting happiness and contentment.

1. Embracing Support and Community

The power of community and support often enhances the path toward positive body image and sexual fulfillment. On the way to a positive body image and sexual fulfillment, plus-sized communities and support groups are invaluable resources. Together, these resources create a foundation of strength, encouragement, and togetherness through empowering shared experiences, participation in body-positive communities, online forums, professional-led seminars, local support groups, inclusive fitness communities, and social media advocacy. Plus-sized people can negotiate their journey with resilience by accepting the support these communities give, creating a sense of community that celebrates their bodies and encourages a healthy and productive sexual life.

Now, let's emphasize the value of plus-sized communities and support groups, which offer a platform for empowerment, encouragement, and the sharing of experiences.

Sharing Experiences to Empower:
Plus-sized support groups are powerful environments where members can draw strength from one another's experiences. People facing comparable obstacles can talk about shared worries, share thoughts, and give helpful counsel. This shared understanding strengthens the bonds between people, lessening feelings of loneliness and laying the groundwork for healthy sexual and self-image.

Communities that Value the Body:
Getting involved in body-positive communities is essential to developing a positive outlook. These communities encourage self-love, question social conventions, and celebrate variety. Places that promote plus-sized bodies can provide comfort to plus-sized individuals by creating an atmosphere that supports self-assurance and a positive self-perception of their individual beauty.

Internet Discussion Boards for Protected Expression: Online forums offer plus-sized people in the digital era a secure and convenient venue to express themselves. Without fear of criticism, these forums encourage candid discussions about relationships, sexual encounters, and body image. People are encouraged to discuss their successes and struggles in online places, which fosters a helpful virtual community.

Local Support Teams:
For plus-sized people, there is a real sense of community provided by local support

organizations. These organizations frequently arrange get-togethers, courses, or events where people can interact in person. Deeper relationships can be made in the intimate setting of local support groups, which promotes a sense of community and encouragement from one another.

Expertly Guided Workshops:
Expert-led workshops created especially for larger-framed people provide focused direction and knowledge. Subjects including body positivity, accepting oneself, and developing a satisfying sexual life may be discussed in these sessions. These expert-led seminars offer a complete approach to help by fusing the camaraderie of a group setting with the insights of experts.

Communities for Inclusive Fitness and Wellness: Participating in health and fitness communities that are inclusive fosters overall well-being. These communities emphasize health and self-love by encouraging physical activities that build a positive relationship with one's body. These settings provide plus-sized people with a safe haven where they may put their health first and lead active lifestyles.

Advocacy and Representation on Social Media: Social media sites are effective instruments for representation and advocacy. Plus-sized people can draw motivation and encouragement from advocates, campaigners, and influencers who value a variety of body shapes. A more empowered and affirming mindset can be achieved by engaging with and following body positivity advocates.

2. Expert Guidance and Counseling: Promoting Positive Emotional and Sexual Health

Experts that specialize in helping people navigate the nuances of their experiences can frequently add value to the road towards better sexual and emotional well-being. In order to support plus-sized people's positive sexual and mental well-being, expert assistance and counseling is crucial. Counselors play a crucial role in enabling people to embrace their bodies and build happy, rewarding, and emotionally resilient lives by addressing specific difficulties, creating a safe place, navigating intimate relationships, and offering tools for sexual exploration.

This final section acknowledges the critical role that professional assistance and therapy play in helping plus-sized people develop a good outlook, emotional fortitude, and a satisfying sexual life.

Proficiency in Handling Particular Difficulties: Expert advice provides a specific method of tackling the particular difficulties that people who are plus-sized may face. Counselors with training have the understanding and empathy to handle problems with body image, social pressures, and personal fears. Their knowledge guarantees that people get individualized guidance and methods to develop a positive perspective on their bodies and their sexual encounters.

Building a Secure and Compassionate Environment: Through counseling, people who identify as plus-sized can freely express their worries, wishes, and emotional struggles in a safe and accepting environment. A deeper examination of thoughts and feelings is made possible by the counselor-individual relationship that is built on trust in this encouraging setting. Building a foundation for positive emotional well-being requires this trust.

Dealing with Self-Esteem and Body Image: In professional coaching, body image and self-esteem are major areas of concern. Together, clients and counselors confront unfavorable views, encourage self-acceptance, and cultivate a good self-image. People can develop emotional resilience and approach their sexual experiences with confidence by addressing these fundamental issues.

Handling Close Relationships:
In order to help plus-sized people manage romantic relationships, counselors are essential. Professional assistance facilitates the development of healthy and meaningful relationships by addressing communication issues, building empathy within partnerships,

and offering tools for strengthening emotional connection.

Techniques for Communication and Sexual Exploration: Specialists in the domain of sexual counseling provide insightful approaches to sexual inquiry and discourse. They help people navigate possible obstacles in a sexual relationship, express their desires, and create boundaries. Plus-sized people can approach their sexual experiences with confidence and successful communication when they use these tactics.

Including Coping Mechanisms and Mindfulness:.Counselors frequently include coping mechanisms and mindfulness in their counseling. These resources aid in the management of stress, anxiety, and unfavorable thought patterns. Mindfulness has been shown to be especially helpful for plus-sized people in developing a positive outlook and enhancing mental well-being, which can lead to a more fulfilling sexual life.

Extended Assistance and Individual Development: Seeking professional assistance can provide enduring support and opportunities for personal development. Frequent counseling sessions offer a stable environment in which people can examine their changing goals, emotions, and thoughts. This continuous assistance fosters personal development in a variety of spheres of life, including sexuality, and adds to long-term emotional well-being.

Conclusion:

Navigating Pleasure and Well-Being for Plus-Sized Individuals

We explored the many facets of fostering enjoyment and wellbeing for plus-sized people in our exhaustive review. Every chapter provided fresh perspectives that helped readers gain a comprehensive grasp of the potential and difficulties involved in leading a satisfying sexual life. Let's review the main points from each section:

I. Understanding the Intersection of Sexuality and Obesity: Initially, we recognized the significance of comprehending the relationship between sexuality and obesity. Understanding the subtleties of this intersection paves the way for a more in-depth investigation of happiness and wellbeing.

II. Defining the Exploration of Personal Connections: The need of redefining and investigating personal connections for people with plus-sized bodies was emphasized in this section. By highlighting the idea that everyone deserves happy relationships, it established the foundation for an optimistic and welcoming attitude.

III. Social Challenges and Stereotypes: Next, we discussed the societal obstacles and prejudices that overweight people must deal with in relation to happiness and sex. By taking on these difficulties head-on, we hope to promote a better comprehension of the outside influences that might affect a person's well-being.

IV. Understanding Sex and the Overweight: The investigation proceeded by highlighting the significance of comprehending sex and the overweight and urging people to accept their bodies, unique experiences, and wants without passing judgment.

V. Navigating Happiness for Plus-Sized Individuals: This part emphasized the importance of attitude changes and positive self-talk in promoting well-being, with an emphasis on developing self-confidence and resistance against social constraints.

VI. Exploring the Best Sex Positions: A thorough analysis of the ideal sex positions for people of plus-size bodies placed a focus on eradicating preconceptions, addressing issues with body image, and encouraging consent and communication. It was emphasized how crucial it is to recognise a range of wishes and offer a thorough reference to a variety of comfortable positions suitable for varying body shapes.

VI. Resources and Support: The last part discussed how important resources and support are. It demonstrated the strength that comes from community and professional help by acknowledging the value of professional guidance and counseling as well as the empowering function of support groups, communities, and various other resources.

This thorough review confirms that happiness and health for plus-sized people have many aspects. The path is complex and includes learning about societal issues, promoting body positivity, managing close relationships, accepting diversity in sex, and getting professional help. Plus-sized people can tackle the challenges with confidence and embrace a healthy sexual life that honors their individuality and well-being by embracing a holistic approach that integrates constructive communication, self-acceptance, and community support.

Starting a path to embrace pleasure and well-being for those who identify as plus-sized calls for a comprehensive strategy that integrates relationships, self-acceptance, and a satisfying sexual life. We have discovered insights intended to promote understanding, demolish preconceptions, and enable people to find their own way to fulfillment through a detailed examination of important aspects.

Recognizing the Intersection: Initially, we agreed that being overweight and having sex interact. This fundamental insight established the framework for a more in-depth investigation, acknowledging that happiness and wellbeing are intricately linked facets of a person's existence.

Redefining Intimate Relationships: Throughout our investigation, there was a recurring theme regarding the need to redefine personal relationships for people who are plus-sized. By challenging social norms and highlighting everyone's intrinsic worth in the search of happy relationships, it promoted an inclusive viewpoint that promotes healthy connections.

Managing Social Challenges: By exploring societal issues and prejudices, we came face to face with outside forces that have the potential to affect a person's wellbeing. Our goal in confronting these issues head-on was to enable people to defy society norms and confidently accept their bodies and aspirations.

Comprehensive Knowledge of Sexuality and Obesity: Knowledge of sexuality and obesity served as a pillar for our investigation. We wanted to encourage a positive outlook and self-acceptance by emphasizing the value of accepting one's physique, wants, and distinctive experiences without passing judgment.

Developing Self-confidence and Resilience: Overcoming social expectations to maintain happiness was a challenge for plus-sized people. This section encouraged people to build a strong foundation for well-being by highlighting the transformational potential of positive self-talk and mindset alterations.

Examining Ideal Sexual Positions: This in-depth analysis of ideal sexual positions for people with plus-sized bodies attempted to challenge preconceived notions, deal with issues related to body image, and encourage consent and communication. The focus on recognizing varied preferences and offering an extensive manual of various, cozy postures designed for various body types underscored the importance of inclusivity in intimate relationships.

Resources and Support: The importance of resources and support was emphasized in the concluding section. Acknowledging the value of professional advice and counseling, in addition to the empowering function of communities, support groups, and other resources, demonstrated the strength that comes from a sense of community and professional help.

In summary, the book encourages plus-sized individuals to embrace their bodies, have satisfying sexual lives, and have a holistic approach to relationships. This all-encompassing strategy includes accepting a range of relationships, encouraging bonds, questioning social standards, developing self-acceptance, and negotiating close relationships with assurance and openness.

Celebrating Individual Uniqueness: Individuals can start a journey towards enjoyment and well-being that honors their bodies and wants by embracing their uniqueness and fostering an inclusive community. An all-encompassing attitude to fulfillment is encouraged by the calls to demolish prejudices, promote constructive self-talk, and look for professional and community support. These calls together make a harmonic chorus.

Empowered Navigation: This thorough investigation empowers plus-sized people by offering a roadmap for overcoming social obstacles, embracing self-acceptance, and cultivating deep connections. People can create a meaningful sexual life that fits their goals and objectives by navigating their own road to pleasure and well-being with an emphasis on positivity, inclusivity, and making educated decisions. By doing this, we declare that regardless of societal norms or physical characteristics, everyone has the right to happiness, fulfillment, and connection, regardless of societal expectations or body size.